SMALL
STEPS
BIG
CHANGE

Radical
Rest

Note from the author

This book is not meant to be a one-size-fits-all solution. I want you, the beautiful, powerful, smart and canny human that you are, to find the bits that work for you and use them. Use them until they don't work, or until something better comes along.

If something here doesn't work for you, awesome! You've learned about yourself. This is true power.

I believe that everything I have shared here is true and has been backed up by science and good practice. The world changes and life changes.

If you decide to take a new supplement or change your exercise routine, please check with your doctor first, especially if you take regular medication or have a chronic health condition. I am a medical professional, but I'm not *your* medical professional, so please be sure to take responsibility for what you put into your body and what you do with it.

Radical Rest

GET MORE DONE BY DOING LESS

Richard Lister

Hardie Grant

BOOKS

Contents

04

Resting To Repair

05

Resting To Renew

06

Resting For Resilience

Conclusion: Start Your Rest Revolution

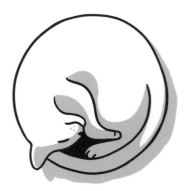

Introduction

Rest. We've been led to believe that it's quite the indulgence: doing nothing, when there's a never-ending list of things that need to be done. Rest is something that you only get to do when all the things on the list are done, right?

WRONG. Rest *is* radical. And I'm not just saying that because I teach and share the principles of *Radical Rest*.

We live in a hectic, busy, technology-driven world. We have mobile phones, tablets and computers, all beeping and demanding our attention 24 hours a day. We have pressure at work, deadlines to meet and projects to complete. We have families to look after and communicate with (something most of us feel like we're failing at every day). We have never-ending to-do lists and lives that we long to live fully, but all of these stresses and strains of modern living are creating unease, pain and discomfort in our minds, our bodies and our psyches. These problems manifest as stress, trauma, depression and/or anxiety, low sex drive, fertility issues, menstrual health issues, a lack of sleep, a lack of energy – a lack of pretty much everything.

Some people manage the symptoms with prescription drugs; others turn to marijuana and gin, while others look to plant-based medicine and entheogens to help 'take the edge off'.

In a society where, right now, it's seen as a revolutionary act to be happy, it's clear that we need a new approach. We need *Radical Rest*. Radical rest is the antidote to a highly pressurised, fear-filled, technological age.

I'm writing this during the coronavirus pandemic of 2020, a time when many people around the world have been forced to pause; a time when it has become clear that the old systems – the ones that had us all living at super-fast speed, in a constant state of 'doing', working long hours, reacting rather than responding, and experiencing burnout, anxiety and depression – are no longer working.

This enforced pause has been a global reminder that rest is, indeed, radical.

The act of slowing down, making the time and space to simply 'be' rather than 'do', allows our bodies to reset, recharge and harmonise with the natural rhythm of nature. My wish is that, in this sacred global pause, we will recognise and remember why rest *is* radical. When we rest, we heal. Our immunity increases, our resilience grows, anxiety and depression are reduced, and recovery is possible.

Rest *is* essential.

01

·

What is Rest & Why is it Radical?

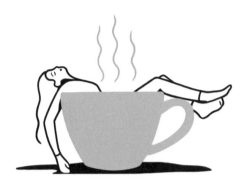

A Self-care Resource

Rest is when you stop 'doing' and allow your body and system time to recover and repair. It's something you can, and absolutely should, schedule into your day and life. It's your most potent self-care resource and needs to be something we respect and value as a way to manage and maintain our human energy system.

Rest lets us unplug from the relentless demands of the nine-to-five work pattern. This pattern often means we're abruptly woken from our natural rest and restorative sleep pattern by an alarm, which

13

ultimately impacts how we experience the day and manage our energy. When we are jarred awake like this, our bodies start the day stressed and on the lookout. Our emotions are automatically more strained, all because we woke ourselves up with a shock.

For many of us, as soon as the alarm goes off in the morning, we are in a rush; we're not present in our bodies. This can lead to us making poor decisions about life, love and everything else throughout the day. And yet we keep doing it. We are caught in this loop because we've been taught that everything that is worthwhile is *outside* ourselves: so we strive, work hard, tick off all the achievements and make money to buy things. In doing so, we further solidify the idea that anything of value is *outside* ourselves, and that everything *inside* ourselves is worthless.

This is why making time for rest is radical, because when you lie down and rest, you stop: you pause, you create space in your system and you recognise what's *actually* important. (Clue: your own inner wisdom. Except you've rarely been still and quiet for long enough to hear it.)

This book is a reminder that, when faced with information overload, along with high levels of stress, anxiety and burnout, rest is necessary.

Radical Rest is a collection of dynamic tools, practices, prescriptions and suggestions that you can tailor to meet your needs. These tools are for everyone, from all walks of life and any belief system. You'll find that they are often built upon medical science, cutting-edge neuroscience and ancient yogic and Ayurvedic practices.

I'm a registered Nurse, and evidence-based practice is my jam.
If I can't back it up, it's not in here. I'm also a health and feel-better
Coach, Master NLP (neuro-linguistic programming) practitioner,
TRE (Tension, Stress and Trauma Release) practitioner, integrated
health and rehab specialist, yoga teacher, massage therapist and
Ayurveda practitioner. I have worked in the NHS for more than fifteen
years, most of which I have spent in the accident and emergency
department.

I experienced a breakdown back in 2013, which led me to study
alternative health care. I discovered that rest is radical, so I now work
with my feet firmly in both camps, meaning I'm able to provide a
holistic approach to healthcare and wellness.

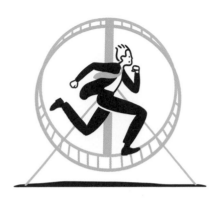

Radical Rest
is Not Sleep

Of course, we need sleep. But radical rest is *not* sleep. It's how you get the best from your body by ensuring that the living, biological systems you were born with work in the best way possible. You can do this by mitigating and managing the stress you experience.

"When we're stressed, we can't rest."

We live in an environment that is overloading us with information. Our whole world is set up to be productive. We even measure the values of our countries by their Gross Domestic Product (GDP): in other words, the money they produce. This is a symptom of how our culture has evolved: more productivity, more stuff, more creation, more stimulation.

This is great for the bottom line in business, but it's not so good for the human experience.

Right now, we've got the highest ever recorded levels of anxiety and stress. Eighty-five to ninety-five per cent of US doctors' appointments are stress-related; people are burning out left, right and centre; and being overwhelmed is starting to cause chronic health problems.

Here are some figures from people in the US and UK:
- Eighteen per cent of adults experience anxiety.
- Fifty-five per cent of adults experience stress.
- Twenty-three per cent of adults experience burnout.
- Sixteen per cent of women and thirteen per cent of men experience being overwhelmed.

These numbers mean that it's highly likely that you, a colleague or a relative are currently experiencing a stress-related symptom.

We are creatures of survival. We have evolved over hundreds of millions of years to be here, right now. We have bodies that are ready to hunt, fight or run. These bodies are meant to experience transient stress: stress that comes and goes. We are not designed to spend all day sitting in a cubicle or scrolling through our phones and experiencing constant, chronic stress.

Constant exposure to stress in any form is simply not good for our bodies. We are not designed to be constantly producing, doing and acting – we need time to integrate, to relax, to process, to rest.

Did you know, offices are one of *the* worst spaces to be creative in? Think about it. We go to the office, we sit in our little box and our unconscious mind starts worrying about all the things around us: the judgements, the expectations, the obligations, all the things we 'should' do. This gets in the way of our ability to think creatively.

Have you ever noticed that you are at your most creative when you are in the shower, when you're nice and warm and just enjoying the moment. This is because your body is relaxing. This means you are then able to start processing the information in your mind without worrying about that guy three desks over playing his music too loudly.

When your body is resting, when you allow your biological functions to relax and just go 'Aaaaaaahhh', you get out of your own way.

What's that? 'Taking time for yourself to rest is lazy'? We've all heard that before. Our culture has conditioned all of us to believe that we are only useful if we are doing and producing. (I believe women experience this slightly more than men due to our social conditioning: women are judged even more harshly when they take time for themselves #patriarchysucks.) But what we've forgotten is that this constant push for productivity is not the way we have evolved. We are creatures that use stress to win, but then we need to rest in order to be productive again.

We have evolved to get stressed in order to give us the energy and adrenaline we need to escape a threat. We run away from the tiger, then we allow ourselves to rest and recover once we are safe.

But in the modern world, we don't do that. When we leave the office at the end of a work day, we don't have time to recover from the 'tiger'. Work emails come through to our phone; we've got to rush to get to our date for the next appointment; we need to phone our parents; we want to update social media. All this stress without respite means our bodies never get the chance to heal, to process, to integrate – to rest.

In fact, instead of resting, we are encouraged to numb ourselves instead: to buy the thing, eat the cookies, drink the wine. The two sensations may feel similar to begin with. Numbing gives you the chemical hit your body wants and stops you from having to feel the negative emotion that you're trying to escape. You probably feel a (temporary) positive emotion when you initially pacify yourself with the wine/cookies/material purchase but, ultimately, it doesn't leave you feeling restored. Eating a load of chocolate or bingeing on a series of your favourite show may feel like resting, but it's not (although we'll explore how it can be used as rest later). We've been trained, programmed and hypnotised to believe that we are resting when what we are actually doing is consuming. When we numb, we don't get the healing and the integration that rest provides. This means we continue to numb some more, and so the cycle continues.

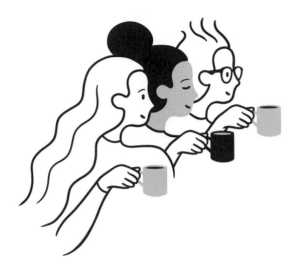

Be Revolutionary: Rest

- When we rest, we become more vital.
- When we rest, we become more creative.
- When we rest, we heal and fight disease.
- When we rest, we regenerate.
- When we rest, we reduce our levels of stress and anxiety.
- When we rest, we are able to learn better.
- When we rest, we become better.

Who wouldn't want some of *that* secret sauce?

There is no blame or shame in this book. You, me, everyone – we are all doing the absolute best we can with the tools we have. If you weren't, you wouldn't be here, reading this book.

Right now, you are doing amazingly well: perfectly, in fact. You're here because we can make choices to do things differently when we learn more.

You don't have to go to medical school or put on a leotard and stand on your head to learn these things. You just have to read this book and practise the things that feel right to you.

Think about learning to walk. The first step you ever took was probably not pretty or easy. Of course, you won't remember it, but go and search the internet for 'babies falling over' and you'll see what I mean. All those little people are learning a new thing. As part of that learning, they fall. And you will too as you learn the techniques in this book. It doesn't matter if you don't do them perfectly; as long as you keep trying, they *will* work.

I want to help you cultivate a relationship with rest, one that is sustainable and transformative. So, take a deep breath in, and let it all out on the exhale. You are amazing. Right here, right now.

Let's get radical. Let's rest.

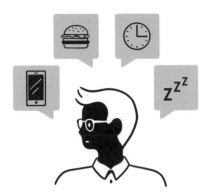

Quiz: How to Tell if you Need to Rest

Notebook time, people. Answer the questions below:

1. Have you yawned in the last two hours? Yes/No
2. Was your last pee more than two hours ago? Yes/No
3. Is feeling stressed a normal experience for you? Yes/No
4. Did you use your phone or tablet in bed last night? Yes/No
5. Do you eat a lot of processed food? Yes/No
6. Do you work nine-to-five? Or shifts? Yes/No
7. Do you feel like you need a nap in the afternoon? Yes/No

Results

If you answered mostly Yes: you need more rest.

If you answered mostly No: you *may* need more rest.

Personally, I think *everyone* needs more rest.

02

·

The Science
of Rest

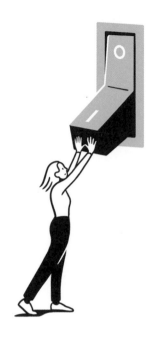

Why is Rest So Hard to Come By?

Radical rest gives us the ability to rest ourselves on every level: mind, body and spirit. It means we can rest not just one part, one system, one function of ourselves, but *all* of them. Before we can begin to improve the many ways in which we can rest, we first need to understand more about it. Why do we need rest, and why can it be so hard to come by?

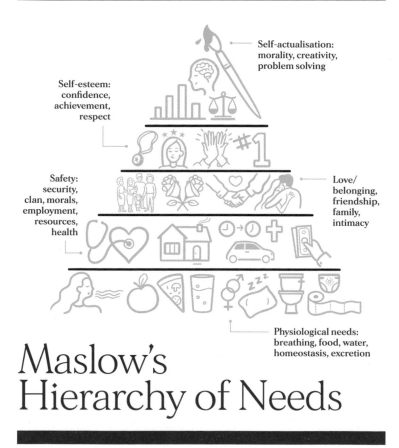

Self-actualisation:
morality, creativity,
problem solving

Self-esteem:
confidence,
achievement,
respect

Safety:
security,
clan, morals,
employment,
resources,
health

Love/
belonging,
friendship,
family,
intimacy

Physiological needs:
breathing, food, water,
homeostasis, excretion

Maslow's Hierarchy of Needs

Radical rest is based on several principles, one of which is Maslow's hierarchy of needs.

Abraham Harold Maslow was an American psychologist and the creator of a theory known as 'Maslow's hierarchy of needs'. This theory is based around the idea that good psychological health requires the fulfilment of certain innate human needs, in order of priority, culminating in self-actualisation.

Each level of this pyramid shows us what we need in order to survive and feel fulfilment. At the bottom of the pyramid are the things we need to actually survive from day to day; at the top is what we need in order to feel fulfilled. Each need level has to be met before you can move on to the next: it's no good being morally fulfilled if you don't have any water to drink – you'll die. The other levels of the pyramid include safety, social belonging and esteem, finishing with self-actualisation at the top.

Radical rest works in the same way. When our needs are met, our bodies and minds relax, allowing us to rest effectively. We can rest through food, drink, sleep, sex, hugs, ideas, community or morality (to name a few). By making sure that we rest radically, from the bottom of the pyramid up, we can make sure that we are healthy in all parts of our lives. This is what radical rest is all about: not focusing on just one aspect of ourselves, but paying attention to the whole picture. When we allow what is going on around us, and the idea of what we 'should' be doing, to get in the way of meeting our own needs, we start to build stress into our bodies. Making, really good nourishing rest nigh-on impossible.

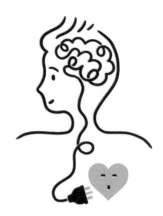

Neuroscience for the Win

"The body feels emotion."

DEEPAK CHOPRA

Our bodies are old – like, 200,000 years old. Not individually – that would be weird – but in terms of versions. We are still working with Human Body version 1: version 2.0 is not even on the cards yet. While we still don't *completely* understand how our bodies work, we do have a pretty good idea.

One of the key things to understand as we move forward is that our minds and bodies are not separate, they are intrinsically connected. Right now, at this moment, think of your favourite food; the scent of it, the taste of it, the feel of it in your hands and its texture in your mouth as you chew. Is your mouth watering? Do you feel hungry? Your mind made your body respond. This is a crude and simple example of the mind–body connection.

Pavlovian reflex

A good example of this mind–body connection is Pavlov. (Not pavlova – that is a dessert and, while it's yummy, they are two different things.) No, Pavlov: you know, the guy who rang bells when his dogs ate?

"Life is really simple, but we insist on making it complicated."

CONFUCIUS

Pavlov decided he wanted to test his theory that dogs would salivate when they saw food. He used a straw in the dogs' mouths to measure their saliva as they waited impatiently for their dinner. After a few days, Pavlov noticed that the dogs would start to salivate when they heard the footsteps of the assistant on their way to feed them. So, he conducted an experiment where the dogs heard the sound of a bell before they were fed. Eventually the dogs would salivate whenever they heard the bell, even without food present. Pavlov realised that the physiological response to the idea of being fed still took place, even if the pup did not actually get to eat anything.

When you see an advert for your favourite food, you may notice
that you are salivating as your mouth gets ready to eat. Another
example is the way that your heart starts beating faster when you
see someone you love. This is your mind's response to a stimulus
causing a physical reaction in the body. And it's a two-way street.
What happens within our bodies, and what happens to them, affects
our minds.

All of this tends to be completely unconscious: after all, it's super
hard to make yourself salivate or itch or get horny. Our unconscious
minds control all the bits of our bodies that you don't have to
think about, such as heart rate, digestion, defecating or sweating.
Technically, this is the Autonomic Nervous System, or ANS.

Our bodies are controlled by our brains via the ANS. Our nervous
system travels all over the body and controls movement, sensation
and bodily functions. If we control, consciously, something our
bodies do, a response is activated in the unconscious mind. You
can demonstrate this now: try breathing in and out, fast, through
your mouth for a minute, then feel your heart rate. The change is
your ANS realising you are breathing fast and so increasing your
heart rate to get ready for some action.

For our purposes, the ANS is broken down into two subsystems,
the Parasympathetic Nervous System (PNS) and the Sympathetic
Nervous System (SNS). The PNS is the 'rest and digest' system: it's
concerned with making sure you are calm and relaxed, that you're
able to heal from injuries and digest food, and that you get some

good-quality sleep. The SNS is the battle-stations system. It's there
to get stuff done. It's often known as the Fight, Flight or Freeze
System (there is a fourth F, mating, but that is for another book).
Here, I'm going to refer to the SNS as the Fight or Flight System,
and the PNS as the Rest and Digest System.

Without the Fight or Flight System, all we would do is eat chips on
the sofa and watch reruns on Netflix. The Fight or Flight System is all
about action. Need to run for the bus? Fight or Flight System. Need
to get to the crowded bar? Fight or Flight System. Need to lift weights
at the gym? You got it: Fight or Flight System. It's extremely useful –
when we need to take action. The problems start when the switch for
the Fight or Flight System is stuck in the 'on' position because we've
been exposed to an excess of stimulation. This is what happens
when we experience stress, burnout, PTSD or being overwhelmed.

The purpose of the Fight or Flight System is to keep us safe.
When our mind tells us we are not safe, whether that's because
there's a rampaging tiger outside or because someone on social
media is talking trash about us, the Fight or Flight System switches
to 'on'. And when it's on, we find it hard to get the rest we need.
It's hard to rest when we are not feeling safe, because our bodies
think we are about to be attacked. What's important here, though,
is that both scenarios create the same response in our bodies:
the rampaging tiger is equal to the social media drama, and the
same hormones and neurotransmissions are released. That's how
we're wired. Our nervous systems are effective – but, sometimes,
they're also a bit dumb.

"We have two states: Fight or Flight and Rest and Digest. Moving between the two is natural. Getting stuck in one causes problems."

Every system in the body is linked to the ANS, and therefore gets stimulated or deactivated according to what the ANS is doing. This is when we start to get long-term problems associated with not resting properly. When we get over stimulated by things we can't or won't action, be they real tigers or metaphorical ones, we can get overwhelmed, become anxious or depressed, experience burnout or develop medical conditions linked to stress.

When we get stressed, we release a hormone called cortisol, which makes our liver release energy from storage. This extra energy floods our muscles, getting us ready to run or fight. Great if there's a real-life tiger coming to eat you; not so great if the problem is actually a social media drama. For the tiger, we actually *need* the extra energy. For the social media fall-out, we don't. We just need a mute switch.

In order to rest, we must first work out how to manually switch off our Fight or Flight response so that we can Rest and Digest. As I mentioned earlier, one of the great things about our nervous system is that it is not a one-way street. It doesn't just send orders from the mind to the body: it can also send orders from the body to the mind.

Because the nervous system is unconscious, we can't easily control it. But what we can do is influence bodily functions that then have an effect on the nervous system. This is the clever bit.

To experience deep, restorative rest, we can use our bodies' natural processes to help us drop into rest and relaxation mode. To reach our Rest and Digest Systems, we need to utilise our bodies' secret pathways. One way of doing this is through our breathing. When we breathe in and out through the nose, our bodies naturally recalibrate to the Rest and Digest System. It's been done for thousands of years by yogis in India, and it's now practised all over the world.

This next concept is a fun one, and one you can look at in yourself with relative ease. We are not just humans: we are billions of years of development in a raincoat pretending to be humans. This means that our biology and neurology have developed from different influences, and these influences can be seen in the way that our brains work. We have a very primitive brain function simply wants to keep us alive – that means being fed and watered, and not being eaten: this is our squid brain. We have another, more modern layer: this is the monkey brain. The monkey brain layer has all the social survival bits built into it. It knows emotions, and socialising, and some simple problem-solving. This brain is what gets stressed when we are on our own. Finally, we have the most recent layer (and by recent, I mean, like, 40,000 years ago recent). This part of our brain can reason, think and plan. It remembers. It can build complex reasoning patterns and send rockets to the Moon, as well as develop Furbees. This is the human brain that makes us *us*. To access your squid brain, go to the supermarket when you are hungry and see what you buy: that's your squid brain in action. When you feel afraid of the dark, or experience FOMO, that's is your monkey brain. And the human brain has all the anxiety and depression, plus creativity and inspiration. Clever us, right?

Breathing exercise: Square breathing

Special forces soldiers in war zones use this technique. In fact, it was taught to me by soldiers that I was training in the emergency department. This is how you do it:

- ◆ Begin by slowly exhaling, emptying all the air out of your lungs.
- ◆ Now gently inhale, through your nose, for a slow count of four.
- ◆ At the top of the breath, hold for a count of four.
- ◆ Gently exhale, through your mouth, for a count of four.
- ◆ At the bottom of the breath, pause and hold for a count of four.

Use this technique whenever you are feeling even slightly stressed. You can do this anytime, anywhere, but I'd suggest not doing it while driving (purely because it relaxes you so much).

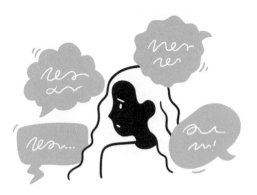

Societal
Hypnosis

There's a psychological element to rest, too, which we briefly explored on pages 19 and 20. We've all been conditioned to believe that production is the most important thing in the world: that making more, and consuming more, is what we are actually here for. This is not actually a truth. I like to call this societal hypnosis. It's what we've been trained, influenced and hypnotised to believe. Seven billion people can't be wrong ... or can they? What if, instead of striving to produce more and consume more, we were to strive to be happier? What if, in order to do that, we took a breath? What if, instead of rushing to read that text message straight away, we allowed it to go unread for a few minutes, what if we waited until we were present? Would the world end? Or, would our experiences actually be better?

"You are the writer, producer, and director of your own mind programmes."

ELIZABETH BOHORQUEZ, RN

Breathing exercise: Two-minute rest
Perhaps eight minutes is too long to begin with. Let's try two minutes.

- Set your phone's timer to two minutes. That's 120 seconds. Now turn the phone over so that you can't see the screen.
- Inhale through your nose and hear the sound it makes. (If you're all bunged up, you can use your mouth.)
- Hold your breath for a count of two.
- Now exhale through your mouth. Hear the sound (a bit like Darth Vader). Hold, with your lungs empty, for a count of two.
- Repeat until the alarm goes off, concentrating on the sound of your breath. If you find yourself getting distracted, focus on the sound of your breath.

Congrats: you've just practised resting for two minutes. That's 0.001 per cent of your day. Has the world ended? You've also just used your breath to regulate your nervous system, as we discussed on pages 42 and 43. You've rested and allowed your body to restore itself a little. To rest radically, we need to make our bodies, minds and spirits take a breath and switch states, enabling us to reach a calm, restful place.

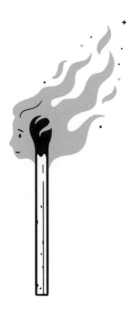

Inflammation

Inflammation is one of the natural responses your body has to stress. It happens because, if you are wounded, you will bleed less if your tissues are inflamed. Think about the last time you cut yourself, the way that the wound got red and swollen? That's inflammation.

But, as we've already discussed with the roaming tiger, this response is not so valuable when the thing your body is reacting to is not an acute physical threat or challenge, but an argument online or a legal case that's dragging on. In these cases, rather than helping your body, inflammation can become a chronic condition.

"It's not stress that kills us; it is our reaction to it."

HANS SELYE

SMALL STEPS: REDUCING INFLAMMATION

Recent research by some clever folks in Berkeley, California, has shown a mechanism that works to reduce inflammation. It is found in fish oil, which contains omega-3 fatty acids. The anti-inflammatory molecules are called specialised pro-resolving mediators (SPMs), and they have a powerful effect on white blood cells, as well as controlling blood vessel inflammation.

All of that is a super-complex way of saying this: 'Take fish oil capsules daily. They will reduce your chronic inflammation and improve brain health.'

Remember to always check with your doctor before starting new supplements. Also, if you are allergic to fish, fish oil capsules are not your friend.

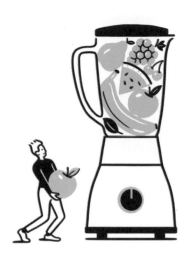

Antioxidants

"My approach is to start from the straightforward principle that our body is a machine. A very complicated machine, but nonetheless a machine, and it can be subjected to maintenance and repair in the same way as a simple machine, like a car."

AUBREY DE GREY

As I've explained, when we are exposed to situations that stress us, our bodies respond with set chemical reactions, hormones and neurotransmitters. One of these responses is called oxidative stress, which means that the level of oxygen radicals in our bodies interferes with the workings of our cells.

Oxygen radicals are unstable oxygen molecules that easily interact with other molecules and basically cause trouble. So, a bit like a mob of people carrying pitchforks and flaming torches, they wind up the other molecules and cause chaos. They smash shopfronts, throw bricks and generally interfere with how your cells are working. Remember in biology at school, we learned that 'the mitochondria are the powerhouse of the cell'? Well, oxygen radicals interfere with this powerhouse.

How do we stop this? In the same way as we stop the pitchfork-carrying, torch-bearing mob. We send in a force to neutralise them: antioxidants.

When it comes to oxygen radicals, antioxidants are like your body's bouncers. I'm sure you've seen what happens when there's trouble and bouncers get involved. Remember that pricey smoothie you drank the other day? The antioxidants it contained will stop these radicals and the damage they're doing.

So, what's this got to do with rest? It's simple: to effectively rest, we've got to stop the stress. So that smoothie is actually helping your body to de-stress and relax. By managing how our cells respond on a metabolic level, we allow ourselves to repair and recover: not just from day-to-day stuff, but from injuries and disease.

The good news is you don't need an expensive smoothie to provide antioxidants. You can get them in plenty of other ways.

Good sources of specific antioxidants include:

* allium sulphur compounds – leeks, onions and garlic
* anthocyanins – aubergines (eggplants), grapes and berries
* beta-carotene – pumpkins, mangoes, apricots, carrots, spinach and parsley
* catechins – red wine and tea
* copper – seafood, lean meat, milk and nuts
* cryptoxanthins – red capsicum, pumpkins and mangoes
* flavonoids – tea, green tea, citrus fruits, red wine, onions and apples
* indoles – cruciferous vegetables, such as broccoli, cabbage and cauliflower
* isoflavonoids – soybeans, tofu, lentils, peas and milk
* lignans – sesame seeds, bran, wholegrains and vegetables
* lutein – corn and green, leafy vegetables, like spinach
* lycopene – tomatoes, pink grapefruit and watermelon
* manganese – seafood, lean meat, milk and nuts
* polyphenols – thyme and oregano
* selenium – seafood, offal, lean meat and wholegrains
* vitamin A – liver, sweet potatoes, carrots, milk and egg yolks
* vitamin C – oranges, blackcurrants, kiwi fruit, mangoes, broccoli, spinach, capsicum and strawberries
* vitamin E – vegetable oils (such as wheatgerm oil), avocados, nuts, seeds and wholegrains
* zinc – seafood, lean meat, milk and nuts
  We'll explore food in greater detail in chapter three.

THE SCIENCE OF REST: RECAP

- Maslow's hierarchy of needs shows that we have different levels of needs that must be met in order for us to thrive. To rest radically, we should rest on every level.
- Our minds and bodies are linked, and what affects one will also affect the other.
- Our Autonomic Nervous System (ANS) can be broken down into two subsystems: the Sympathetic Nervous System (SNS), or the 'Fight or Flight System', and the Parasympathetic Nervous System (PNS), or the 'Rest and Digest System'.
- Our Fight or Flight System keeps us safe when we're under threat, but it can't differentiate between different types of threat, so we have the same physical reaction to a falling-out on social media as we would to being chased by a tiger. This can lead to overstimulation, stress, anxiety, overwhelm and burnout because we get stuck in Fight or Flight instead of moving into Rest and Digest.
- Stress can lead to inflammation.
- Antioxidants can combat the reaction of our bodies to stress and help us recover more efficiently.

03

Resting
to Reset

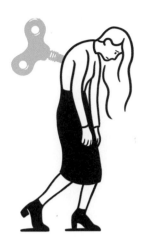

Understanding
Your Body

It's super annoying that we are in these bodies without access to an instruction manual. I mean, even the oven has an instruction manual. (Not that I can work out how to reset the oven clock, even with the manual ... not my greatest analogy.) What I'm saying is that it's hard to figure out how your body works. To make it more complicated, each body is subtly different. What is awesome for your friend may not be awesome for you. Take gluten, for example. I could happily devour a whole bakery (and have); my wife? Not so much. Each human is different. Manual or no manual, what *is* useful to know is that our bodies have the innate ability to shut down and restart.

When we are exposed to lots of stimulation, our minds and bodies can become overwhelmed, even if we don't realise it. Unfortunately, stimulation is addictive to our primitive minds. We LOVE IT. It's a literal drug. The problem is that when we start to over-stimulate, we don't give ourselves the chance to process, so our brain gets fuzzy and our thinking gets disordered. You know that feeling at 4 a.m. when you're still scrolling on your phone? That's the feeling.

It's like when you have too many photos stored on your smartphone. The phone gets slow and sluggish and it takes ages to open your apps. When you reset it, the phone has a little think, a chance to recover, and then it comes back to life with a bit more energy. Now you can delete those 200,000 selfies that are taking up all the memory (no judgement here).

When we rest, we give our bodies, minds and spirits the chance to reset, so we can then process and get rid of our metaphorical 200,000 selfies. This reset enables us to become more efficient and fulfilled.

PERMISSION TO REST

I've already said that we need to rest, yet many of us are under the societal hypnosis to constantly produce, make and do.

So right now, and right here, you, the person reading this,

I encourage you to break the spell:

You are allowed to rest.

You are allowed to take time for yourself.

You are allowed to rest in the way that feels good and nourishing.

You shouldn't need permission, but if you do, consider this your permission slip.

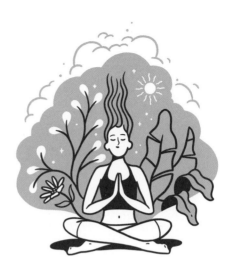

How to Rest

The 'how to' in 'how to rest' is important. It implies action, and we like action. In fact, most of us would rather be doing than thinking. So, let's utilise that and make rest something that we actually *do*, rather than just passively experience. It's much more fun to be involved in stuff than to let it happen around you, right?

Resting can be any activity that lets your body stop being forced to be aware of all the other things that are going on. This means that rest is different for all of us. Rest does not mean sitting still in a dark room or having a nap. Some people need to run around to rest; others need to meditate or watch reality TV. Some people require quiet and solitude in order to relax; others might need to stand in a stadium and scream at the umpire. What is important is that, whatever form it takes, rest should normalise your nervous system, ideally into the 'Rest and Digest' phase (pages 39 and 40).

In order to rest, we need to make sure our bodies and minds feel safe. If they don't feel safe, we can't rest effectively. You need to know your own body's triggers and pathways to rest; they are as unique as you are.

Here is a selection of things that are commonly seen as restful. You can adapt them to suit you.

- Being in nature. Whether you're in the local park or somewhere deep in the Rockies, being in nature helps our bodies relax into the Rest and Digest state. All that matters is that you're somewhere natural.
- Being alone. Spending time alone is a powerful tool. No judgement, no social media, just you. We are programmed to be aware of and respond to the humans around us in order to keep ourselves safe. Being alone allows us to drop that awareness and relax into our own experience. This is an especially useful way to rest if you work in a client-facing job.
- Passive meditation. Passive meditation is where you let something distract you. Listening to the radio or music is great. Or, if you are going to kick it old school, read a book (one that's made of paper, not on your tablet). This allows your brain to consciously focus on something else, and then lets your unconscious sort all the other stuff out. Audiobooks are good for this, as are podcasts that you're

only half-interested in. You could also use TV. The problem with TV, though, is that it's designed to engage you and get all you focus, then try and sell you something. When I use TV for this, it tends to be something I'm already familiar with. *The Lord of the Rings* extended cut marathon, anyone? However, the best tool forpassive mediation, by a long way, is not watching Legolas kill orcs for the hundredth time. It's chants. Yoga chants, Gregorian Chants, Bhakti Yoga ... the list is endless. What chants have that the other tools don't is that they tend to be in a different language, Latin, Hindi, Sanskrit or Gurumukhi, to name a few. This means that your brain can't grab the words as easily as English. (The assumption here is that you don't speak those languages!) Chants also have a repetitive beat, thus giving your conscious mind permission to follow the beat, and the cadence, while your unconscious mind gets on with sorting everything else out.

- Active meditation. This is where you actively choose to meditate. I use yoga or kundalini yoga, actively focusing on the practice, chant or movement. Just as with passive meditation, you choose to focus on one thing, for example your breathing or, in Kundalini Yoga, how much your arms hurt or where your gaze is. This allows your unconscious mind to take over in the background and relax into Rest and Digest.
- Having a warm bath. This allows your body to relax into Rest and Digest mode, as you feel warm and safe. (Ice baths don't count, as your body will go into Fight or Flight mode).

Sports

I mentioned earlier that some people need to run around in order to rest. While activities like paintball or football are stimulating and will technically put you into Fight or Flight mode, ultimately, playing sports is relaxing, because your body is doing what it was designed for: hunting. All sports are a derived from that theme (some are quite well removed). And it's the after-effects of sport that are important. After that stimulation, the body can relax into Rest and Digest mode. Your primal body knows it's done the thing to make sure it's safe: it has fought, hunted, run away or mated, and its biological mechanisms are happy.

Give yourself time

Once the body feels safe, it's time to start making the mind feel safe. We are conditioned and programmed to be constantly active, to always be *doing*, so we need to look at how to satisfy that desire to do, while still resting and relaxing.

One way of doing this is to give yourself a certain amount of time to rest, while satisfying your mind that you will be able to get on with the doing afterwards. Using a timer for this can help you train yourself to accept that it's OK to just watch *Real Housewives* for an hour, then answer your emails, rather than trying to do both at the same time. This means you get some meaningful relaxation going on. Just sitting on the couch, typing away at your emails while women yell at each other on the TV does not count as good resting. Set the timer for twenty minutes, or ten minutes, or forty-five; whatever feels good to you. Start small and work your way up if you need to. Turn the timer on and just enjoy your TV programme. You can do the same for a yoga class, a meditation, a hike in the woods, a sunbathe on the beach, or just to gaze wistfully into the distance. Whatever you want to do, set a time limit, trust your tech to remind you, then get on with your rest.

SMALL STEPS: FINDING OUT WHAT WORKS FOR YOU

Try some different things to see what works for you.

- Go out in nature.
- Take a bath.
- Watch TV.
- Listen to music.
- Spend some time alone.

Start with five minutes on your timer and build it up to what feels good for you: it could be twenty minutes; it could be thirty. Whatever number works for you is the best one.

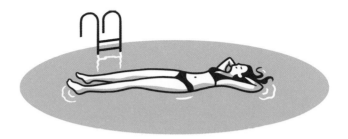

Rest Your Body

Overstimulation

We have an awesome, in-built ability to reset our bodies and minds on a physical level. This is a super-primitive system in our bodies. We can see it in action when animals or people are overloaded with stress and stimulation. You may have experienced it yourself, or seen it happen to friends or loved ones, when something traumatic has happened, like a car crash. The entire body shakes and quivers, but the person is not having a seizure: they are completely aware of what is going on.

While it can look scary and worrying, this shaking is a completely natural process. It happens unconsciously, and we can't consciously stop it, even when it happens at inappropriate times, for example if we have a near miss when driving. So, we tense up and hold on to this overstimulation. Our bodies have evolved to respond to stress in certain ways. These responses might make sense after the extreme example of a car crash above. Where we get into a pickle is when the same pathways get activated when we are sitting in the office and make a mistake.

"The body needs to rest. It needs a lot less exercise than you think."

SYLVESTER STALLONE

When our nervous system gets overstimulated like this, our bodies need to rest so the excess stress can get right out of there. When we don't get the rest we need to process this excess stress, we start to get congestion: a build-up of unprocessed overstimulation that can start to interfere with our normal functions. This can lead to brain fog, poor sleep, poor decision-making, poor focus, to name but a few. There can also be physical symptoms, such as confused digestion (too loose, or too hard) and/or eczema. This is less than ideal.

The psoas muscle and the vagus nerve

Various muscle groups in your body are thought to hold on to this unprocessed overstimulation. One important one is your psoas. This is a sail-shaped muscle at either side of the base of your spine, just above your bum. Author and psoas expert Liz Koch describes the psoas as 'the emotional store of the body'. It is an unconscious muscle; this means that we can't make it move deliberately. It does, however, respond when our unconscious minds need it, usually to stop us from falling over or to stabilise our trunk. It's integral to us being able to walk or sit upright. The psoas tends to get stretched and exhausted when we don't rest and when we let excess stimulation build up in our bodies.

For geeks like me, the psoas is also important because it carries part of the vagus nerve through it. The vagus nerve controls most of our biological functions. It starts in the brain and goes all the way to the pelvis. The psoas and the vagus nerve are connected to the body's memory of stress. This is both awesome and super frustrating. The increase in tension and stress in the psoas stimulates the vagus nerve, which in turn stimulates the stress response all the way up, affecting reproductive organs, the digestive system, the heart and lungs, plus all the endocrine (hormone) making organs. The body then goes into a danger setting, telling the brain, 'Watch out! Danger Will Robinson!'. This is great if there is a tiger: less so if your exhausted psoas is releasing its exhaustion and bringing up a time when you fell off your bike at twelve years old. All that unprocessed stimulation being dumped on you in the middle of the office on a rainy Wednesday afternoon is no fun.

Remember earlier, when I said our biology is a two-way street? (It was, like, in the first chapter: I don't blame you if you forgot.) As a reminder, when our bodies have a response to something, we can use that response to cause a particular reaction. So although we can't consciously make our hearts beat faster, when we tried breathing fast, we saw that our heart rates increased in response.

So ... our psoas and vagus nerve are linked, and we can't consciously activate our psoas to reset our bodies to drop that excess stimulation. This means we have to work out other ways in which we can get the powerful rest needed for our bodies.

I'm sure you're reading this, saying, 'YES! This is me! How do I fix it?' First, you don't need fixing: you are doing awesomely. Second, if you want to help your body rest physically, I can tell you how. I am literally the gift that keeps giving. Remember, rest does not equal sitting on the sofa eating fried chicken, as much as we'd like it too.

The psoas can only be activated unconsciously, either when there is a stressor, or when you are balancing your core, for example if you are in plank position or walking on a narrow path. If we can relax our unconscious control of the psoas, we can release that tension while we consciously rest.

SMALL STEPS: EXERCISES TO REST YOUR BODY

Do these exercises at least three times a day, or preferably every hour when you're at work. Or, if you prefer, just do them as required.

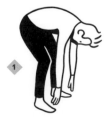

1. Bend forward, making sure you have your knees bent. This will relax your psoas, which plugs into the hamstrings. Slowly count to thirty here or set a timer on your phone for thirty seconds.

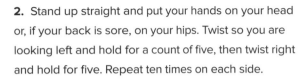

2. Stand up straight and put your hands on your head or, if your back is sore, on your hips. Twist so you are looking left and hold for a count of five, then twist right and hold for five. Repeat ten times on each side.

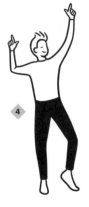

3. Stand up straight, with your hands still on your head (or hips). Push your tummy forward and lean backwards so you feel the stretch along your stomach and pelvis. Repeat at least five times.

Note: If you are double-jointed or hypermobile, when you do this exercise you will need to consciously tense your thighs and tummy and squeeze your pelvic floor as if you are holding on to a wee or doing a Kegel exercise. This will protect your joints and put the load on your muscles.

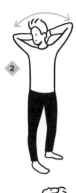

4. Grab your phone and find your favourite dance-about track (I like to use *Jump Around* by House of Pain or *Place your Hands* by Reef, but then I'm old). Turn it up and dance around: let your arms flail; shake your legs, your fingers and your toes; move your jaw and eyes; wiggle your eyebrows. Move it all, however your body wants to move.

Note: If you're going to do this in the office, it's only fair to warn your colleagues in advance. Better yet, get them to join in.

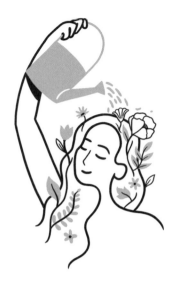

Rest Your Mind

I know, I know. I keep saying that your mind and body are linked, but now I've broken the act of resting down, please remember, this is a two-way street: mind to body, body to mind. Well, that's my prerogative as an author. And please remember, this *is* a two-way street: mind to body, body to mind. This means that resting one helps to rest the other. Let's double down on that and see how we can rest and reset the mind.

When I say reset the mind, I don't mean a total wipe or return-to-factory-settings reset. That would be awkward and embarrassing. I mean getting rid of the congestion and crud that builds up in our minds. This tends to be in the form of unprocessed memories or feelings; songs that loop round and round; ruminating and worrying about staffroom gossip. Whatever it is, it takes up your mental bandwidth and so affects the number of things you can process. To get more out of life, having good mental bandwidth is important. You don't want yours to be jammed up with people behaving foolishly in the staffroom.

"Good friends, good books and a sleepy conscience: this is the ideal life."

MARK TWAIN

The mind is super complex, but by resetting to what is at our core, we can help ourselves to feel better, to manage life with more grace and power, and to generally be awesome. By getting ourselves back into our bodies, we can clear the mental roadblocks in our minds and be sure we have enough bandwidth to move on to the next project.

When we give our minds a finite edge, a start-and-stop point, this enables the mind to relax and stop worrying about things beyond that point. We can do this by focusing on being fully present in our bodies — by consciously inhabiting them. We can reset our minds by reminding them of our bodies. Good, eh?

Have you ever noticed that, the more you have rattling around in your head, the clumsier you get? Or do you find yourself mindlessly eating when you are really busy? This is because you are not fully present in your mind and body. Basically, your mind is so focused on one thing that the body, which doesn't really know what's going on, takes over in the meantime. For example, the body likes chocolate, so, just like a naughty toddler, it happily eats the chocolate while the brain is focusing on the tricky work project.

This disassociation often happens around stressful things, like meeting a new boss, going on a date or giving a presentation. Because the mind is so focused on getting ready for the thing, or looking back at the thing, it forgets to look at where you actually are, and then BANG! You walk into the edge of a table.

We need to make sure that the mind and body are in alignment, to allow the two parts to be together (so they can both enjoy the chocolate/avoid walking into tables). To do this, you need to be *in* your body effectively. This allows you to focus on the here and now and not drift off into whatever ideas you are experiencing.

I'm sure you are after an awesome tool to make this bandwidth-clearing, body-inhabiting magic happen for you – and guess what? You've bought the right book.

SMALL STEPS: EXERCISE TO RESET & REST THE MIND
This is a good exercise for when you are changing pathways at work, for example if you've just had a meeting and now you need to go and be creative, or if you've just been on a site visit and now you need to be super professional and meet the MD to ask for a pay rise.

- Put your headphones on and play a chilled-out track, ideally something without words, or in a language you don't understand. If you want to, set a timer for five minutes on your phone. Otherwise, just go with the flow.
- Put a note on your desk so your colleagues don't interrupt you.
- If you feel comfortable doing so, close your eyes. If not, focus your eyes on something – glittery things like crystals or water work well.
- Take some deep breaths, in through the nose and out through the mouth.
- With each breath, feel the sensations of your body. Feel the air moving over your lips and nose; feel your clothes on your skin; feel the rise and fall of your chest; feel where your bottom touches the chair; feel your fingers; feel where your toes touch your shoes.
- As images come to you, just let them go. Imagine anything that comes to your mind is covered in oil, so that it just slips away.
- Notice what you are smelling; notice what your tummy feels like; notice what your chest feels like; notice what your head feels like.
- Notice where any emotions are. Notice what the emotions feel like: colours, shapes or textures. Let them go.
- Return to your breath.
- When you are ready, open your eyes. Wiggle your fingers and toes, stretch out your arms.

Because I'm awesome, you can download an audio version of this meditation for your phone at *radical-rest.com*, so you don't have to read and meditate at the same time.

Rest electronically

Our minds are programmed to respond to stimulation, which includes all the notifications and adverts that come from our screens, not to mention the blue light. This is great — if you are a marketing company trying to sell toothbrushes, or a business that makes its revenue from clicks. It's not so great for us. Our minds and bodies are not designed to be constantly stimulated in the way that they are with social media, TV, smartphones and computers. The flashy lights and stimulating music you are subjected to as your TV tries to sell you cheese can lead to an excess of stimulation.

"Dynamic activity and deep rest of the mind are complementary to each other."

DEEPAK CHOPRA

Exercising some control over the excess stimulation these electronic tools cause in your brain can give your nervous system a chance to relax back into Rest and Digest mode. By modifying the stimulus our digital environment gives our minds and bodies, we can modify how we release hormones and so rest effectively.

Taking a rest from digital and electronic stimulation will allow our minds and bodies to decompress.

REST YOUR MIND FROM SMARTPHONES

We're going to look at how you can reset your behaviour to help you take a rest from your phone. The goal here is to reset the brain to break the habit of picking up your phone every five minutes to check for notifications.

Do you notice that, when you pick your phone up, your body automatically unlocks it and opens your favourite app? Then, before you consciously realise it, you've checked your emails, looked at your DMs and liked ten posts – all without engaging your conscious mind! This is an example of the development of neuropathways. Our dependence on stimulation causes neuropathways to be formed in the brain, which leads to the creation of behavioural patterns. Essentially, you've become so used to unlocking the phone and opening your favourite app that your conscious brain doesn't even need to be aware of it anymore. It's almost on the level of knowing how to ride a bike or open a can of soda. You don't have to think about it. So, what we need to do is interrupt that behaviour pattern.

SMALL STEPS: BREAK THE SMARTPHONE PATHWAY

Move your favourite app or apps into a folder or off the home screen of your smartphone, so that you actually have to go looking for it rather just having it at your fingertips. Move it again every week. Keep rearranging your screen.

Over a few weeks, this will interrupt the behaviour pattern and break that habit. This is because the established pathway doesn't work: instead, the thumb has to go to another place to open the app, one that it's not trained for. You have to consciously think about it to find the app. This change in pattern allows your brain to re-set, and rest. Turning off the notifications for that app also helps. Our brains are designed to look for new information, and notifications instantly say, 'Look at me, new information here!'. Removing this excess stimulation is an easy victory. We also get to empower ourselves to choose the stimulation, not be passively fed it.

REST YOUR MIND FROM TV

TV companies (and now online streaming platforms) have had decades to hone the art of making you watch, using cliffhangers, mood music and subliminal image placement to keep you hooked. All of these things are designed to get you to watch one more episode, to pay attention to the advertisement, to buy the thing.

One of the elements that is used is blue light. Our brains have evolved to find blue light addictive. It's in sunlight naturally, and it helps our brain make serotonin, a neurotransmitter that wakes us up and helps with a positive mood. Blue lights tells us that we are safe, that we can hunt and that we are alive. The blue light that comes from our TVs stimulates us in the same way. Our brains begin to learn that when we watch this advert with this sound and these colours, we get serotonin and feel good. That makes us want to buy the thing that's being advertised or watch the next episode. Other than turning off the TV, what can we do about this?

SMALL STEPS: BLUE LIGHT-BLOCKING

To rest our minds from this excess of blue light, you can get yourself some blue light-blocking glasses. These glasses have amber-coloured lenses that filter out the stimulating blue light (that's the 450-460nm wavelength, for the geeks out there). This helps interrupt the behaviour patterns we've formed associating the blue light stimulation of the TV with feeling good.

What's also good about these blue light-blocking lenses is that when you use them at your computer during the day, they can help reduce eye strain. This helps to rest your body: another win for you.

Blue light-blocking glasses also help our brains produce melatonin, getting us ready for sleep. Melatonin is a hormone that our brains produce when we are getting less blue light – traditionally, this would have been because the sun had gone down, but our glowing screens keep giving us blue light long after dark. Melatonin is part of the mechanism that allows us to have restful sleep, so blocking the blue light in the lead-up to bedtime can really help.

REST YOUR MIND FROM YOUR COMPUTER

Almost all of us use computers in our work to some extent. Whether we're reading endless email updates from corporate, checking accounts spreadsheets or managing appointments, it's all digital now. What we don't always realise is that everything about our computers is under our control. We can change the colour of the screen. We can make the computer tell us when we've spent too much time on social media or looking at pictures of cats in boxes, or when we've spent hours staring at a spreadsheet trying to work out where the error is.

We are not necessarily addicted to this this sort of stimulation in the same way that we are addicted to our phones (with the possible exception of cats in boxes). It's more that we feel *obliged* to be stuck to our computers at work, as we equate sitting at our computers with being productive. Remember: 'productive' is the buzzword that makes the world go around.

Let's look at how we can address this by resetting our idea of what it is to be productive. Controversially, we need to actually realise that resting at work leads to more productivity.

SMALL STEPS: RESTING AT WORK

The University of California, Berkeley did a study that shows that when we rest at work, our productivity goes up. So, tell your boss you are taking five, and go for a walk. Get outside if you can. Being outside changes your temperature, and your neurological state. There are different smells, different interactions, different experiences for your body, and this allows your nervous system and body to reset, and rest.

The important bit here is to come back to your work once you've decompressed and reset your mind. You should feel refreshed and ready to tackle your work.

Here are some things that can make this easier to achieve:
1. Change your shoes. This is a good life hack for all the time, not just for when you need a break from the screen. Have a pair of shoes that are just for work — don't wear them anywhere else. Put them on when you get to work, and change into your awesome not-work pumps when you leave the building, even if it's just for a walk at lunchtime. This change of shoes helps you change your mental state. Nurses unconsciously use this technique when changing out of their uniforms at the end of a shift. For you, though, it's not so much to avoid taking germs home to your family, it's more to avoid taking your work mindset

home. When you leave your screen, whether it's at the end of the day or just for your quick reset, put those chill-out shoes on.

2. Dance. Move in ways that are not work ways. When you are outside and away from your desk, shake, wiggle, move; do whatever you need to do to make your body feel activated. Do it! Pretend you are in a flash mob (I'm so 2004).

3. Leave work at work. Don't check your emails when you're not at work and try not to think about work outside the office. Podcasts or audiobooks can help if you're finding it difficult to switch off your thoughts about work. They use your conscious mind to process, allowing your unconscious mind to rest.

Quick reset after work

When we finish work for the day, we often don't have a lot of time before the next thing we're supposed to be doing. The mindset and focus required for work is often vastly different from the mindset needed for your improv class, or for an evening in a bar with friends.

Our minds like flowing along processes and patterns that go to known conclusions: habits. This is a useful tool for when we need to do the same thing over and over again. Take commuting: have you ever just arrived at work and realised the last twenty minutes are not in your brain at all? This is because your unconscious mind has taken over the task of getting you to work, by simply doing the same thing it has done multiple times before. What's great about this is that the unconscious mind's most important job is to make sure that you are safe, so as soon as something unexpected happens, your conscious mind takes over. So, if a kid runs past on an amber light, or the person in the car in front slams on their brakes, your conscious mind comes into play and reacts accordingly.

We can use our brain's fondness for patterns to help us reset our minds by creating different patterns with some awesome tools and techniques.

Smells are a primal trigger for us. They go straight to our very primitive brain and trigger things. This is why supermarkets have bakeries onsite and pump the smell of baking bread around the store. That just-baked smell makes us hungry, and so we're more likely to buy more food. Or think about the smell of your childhood home, or wherever you have felt most content. As soon as you smell that scent, your body adjusts to be in the emotional state that you associate with that comforting smell.

Essential oils and oil diffusers are my preferred way to get scent into the air, as burning candles or incense can set off all the fire alarms. Incense is a powerful tool, too, but a smoky one. (I use a supplier who has contacts with the people who actually farm it, so I can be sure it's got good ethics behind it.)

We can use the power of scent to reset ourselves after work, and we can also use it in reverse to get ourselves into work mode.

SMALL STEPS: RESET AFTER WORK
Choose a scent. Essential oils are good for this as they have a strong fragrance, or you can use your favourite perfume, as long as you don't wear that perfume to work. Spray your chosen

scent in the air whenever you leave work to go and meet friends, or when you meet up with them at the at the weekend or on holiday. Basically, every time you see your friends outside work, spray this scent into the air and really breathe it in. Over the period of about three weeks, your brain will begin to associate the smell you've chosen with the idea of chilling with friends. Eventually, you can use this scent to activate your Rest and Digest system.

Exactly the same method can be used to get you into work mode. Choose a different scent (again, either an essential oil or perfume is fine) and spray it in the air just before you walk into work. Once you've sprayed it, deliberately start doing work things. Every time you notice yourself getting right into your work mindset, smell your work scent. Gradually, you'll build the behaviour of going into work mode whenever you smell this particular scent.

You can use this technique for any mental state you want. Going to the gym? Choose a scent as your gym scent. (Lynx body spray, maybe? That's what the gym smells like already. What, just mine? Oh.) Any behaviour can come to be associated with a particular smell. It just takes about three to four weeks to embed, and the more you do it, the stronger it becomes.

RESTING TO RESET: RECAP

◆ Resting gives our minds and bodies a chance to reset. Resting our bodies can rest our minds, and vice versa.

◆ Resting can be any activity that normalises our nervous systems and lets our bodies relax into Rest and Digest mode, from taking a bath to being in nature, meditating or even watching a familiar film.

◆ Setting a timer can help you get used to resting for a specific period of time without worrying about what you 'should' be doing.

◆ The psoas muscle holds on to tension caused by excess stimulation and stress. We can't consciously control the psoas, but by doing certain exercises to relax it, we can release this tension.

◆ Focusing on inhabiting our bodies can help us to rest our minds.

◆ Techniques and tools for interrupting our behaviour patterns around technology like smartphones and TVs can help us reset our habits and rest.

◆ Techniques to reset after work can help us rest more completely and therefore work more effectively.

04

.

Resting
to Repair

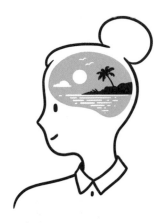

Taking a Break

When looking after people who have been in huge crashes or have heinous injuries, doctors will often put them in a coma. This allows the body to rest, heal and repair. This is especially useful for the brain. While the patient is having this enforced rest, the nurses and doctors will take over their nutrition and hydration needs and look after their other bodily functions, enabling the injured person's body to focus on healing.

When we rest, we allow our bodies to repair and sort out problems. As we have already started to explore in the previous chapter, resting is not just sitting on the sofa in front of your streaming service. Rest can be found in how you eat, drink and recover from a late night.

LISTEN TO YOUR GUT

As a nurse, one of the major metrics I go by with my patients (and myself) is elimination. If you are not having bowel movements or passing urine, there is something going on. Your body is not working properly, and not being rested.

Everyone is different: some people defecate once a day, some people every other day. You will know what is normal for you. If your schedule is off, and you find yourself going more often, or not often enough, you know something is wrong.

To balance your gut, you can look at taking probiotics, getting some extra fibre through things like psyllium husks, and moving more.

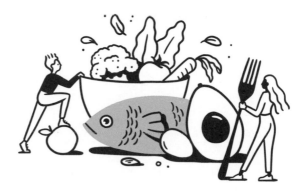

Eating

"Nothing would be more tiresome than eating and drinking if God had not made them a pleasure as well as a necessity."

VOLTAIRE

What we eat – and how we eat it – affects how our bodies process food. Knowing how our bodies will respond to different foods is useful as we can then choose what to eat.

When we eat, our bodies produce a hormone called insulin. Insulin moves the sugar from our bloodstreams and into our cells for storage, keeping our bodies in balance. (My friend Jane has diabetes, which means her body can't produce insulin and too much sugar gets into her blood. This can make her feel rubbish and can cause her to get super sick. People with diabetes may need insulin injections to help their bodies process sugar.) Storing this extra energy in our cells is how we get fat. And guess what, rest fans? Fat causes oxidative stress (page 59), and vice versa. High blood sugar can cause oxidative stress too, a kind of lose/lose situation.

Why am I telling you this? Well, the state we are in when we consume food dictates how our bodies use it. How does food help us to radically rest? We need to make sure that our bodies are as relaxed as possible when we eat. If we eat when stressed, our bodies:

1. **Are not going to digest effectively;**
2. **Will therefore want to store the energy as fat.**

Our bodies can't digest effectively when we're stressed because part of our neurological stress response reduces blood flow to our digestive systems. This is because the digestive system is not essential to life in the short term, but the impact is that it reduces the effectiveness of our digestion. If we consistently eat when stressed, the slowing down of our digestive processes causes imbalances in the bacteria that grow in our digestive tracts, creating more problems still. To rest our digestive systems effectively, we need to look at how we eat.

Get thankful

Here's a cool fact: gratitude reduces stress and moves us into Rest and Digest mode. Our ancestors capitalised on this. They probably didn't do so knowingly (how would 10th-century people know about inflammatory hormones?), but they did practise gratitude when they ate.

They said Grace.

I'm not saying you should spend twenty minutes praying as your mashed potatoes get cold. I'm saying that giving thanks, taking a moment to express true gratitude for the food you are about to eat, is a powerful tool to adjust your state from Fight or Flight to Rest and Digest. This allows your body to effectively process the food you eat. Being in Rest and Digest mode also means that you eat less, as your mind can focus on what you're eating. When we are present and feeling grateful for our food, we eat less and find that we feel fuller, faster. Ohio State University showed this in a meta-analysis in 2015. So it's not only centuries of religious and spiritual practice; modern science says we should be thankful for our food, too.

When stressed, our bodies look for high-energy food that will give us the fuel we need to run or fight. Remember going shopping while hungry? All the carbs, right? What we tend to lack when we are stress-eating is the proteins that our bodies use to repair and grow. Proteins are made up of amino acids, and they are super important to making sure we are healthy.

Practising gratitude before you eat allows you to rest your body and digest effectively. It switches your neurological state from Fight or Flight to Rest and Digest. When we do this, we are able to naturally manage the carbohydrate load we consume, we stop excess cortisol being released, and we turn the amino-acids (the building blocks of our body) into useful tools. Without using fancy words, we are less likely to eat lots of less nutritious food if we are grateful for and present during our meals, and our unconscious brain will pick the foods the body needs first.

SMALL STEPS: GIVING GRATITUDE FOR FOOD

Before I eat, I take three breaths in and out though my nose. This primes my digestion for eating, as smell is a powerful trigger. It also relaxes my nervous system.

I then verbally or internally thank myself for prepping and buying the food, and the food itself for nourishing me. This reduces the production of the stress hormone cortisol in my brain, and lets my body produce some of the good stuff, dopamine, the happy hormone. Gratitude is powerful like that.

I take three more breaths in and out through my nose.

Then I eat.

How we digest our food is also affected by the environment in which we eat. If we sit on the sofa watching TV as we eat, with our bodies squished up and hunched, our digestive tracts are not going to be effective and will get stressed. Sitting up at a table (like actual adult humans) allows our digestive tracts to work effectively.

How to eat restfully

Calorie control and fasting are part of how we've evolved as humans. It's only been in the last hundred years or so that we've had access to such an abundance of food in the world, especially in the West. Before that, during the winter, we would have a restricted calorie intake because there were fewer crops. And as for the idea of three meals a day? This was a 17th-century construct to allow businessmen to network with their colleagues and associates while eating. This led to the creation of the formal lunch.

Nowadays, we have a lot more freedom and can choose how we fuel ourselves. Most food we eat has a known calorie content that we can use to judge how much we're consuming. We know that eating too much causes us to put on weight, and if we are carrying too much fat, we put stress on our heart and lungs. Eating too little puts us into starvation mode, where our bodies start doing weird and not-so-wonderful things like burning muscle and become less efficient at burning energy.

Fasting

Our bodies are designed to survive and, indeed, flourish when there are fewer calories around. In our days as hunter-gatherers, we did not have the option of going to the golden arches when we wanted a snack. Sometimes we got ourselves a woolly mammoth to barbecue; sometimes we got nothing. Our bodies are designed to work in times of plenty and times of famine. To allow ourselves to rest through eating, it's important to look at when we eat, and how much.

Fasting means not eating for a designated period of time, and it is a powerful tool. It allows the body to rest, and it can control the body's drive to store the calories we eat as fat. Fasting allows us to properly process the food we've already consumed and assign it accordingly within the body, rather than getting stressed and overwhelmed by the process. Fasting has been shown to be really effective in supporting the pacification of chronic disease, fat loss and muscle growth.

SMALL STEPS: FASTING AS REST

The 16:8 method

This is one of the most popular intermittent fasting methods. Followers of this method eat all of their calories for the day in an eight-hour window and fast for the remaining sixteen hours of the day. The 16:8 method is popular for beginners because you should be asleep for about half of your sixteen fasting hours.

The 5:2 method

This method involves eating as you normally would for five days a week and eating just 500–600 calories on the other two days. This is another popular method, but many people struggle to avoid bingeing the day after a fasting day.

Eat stop eat

This method that involves a complete twenty-four-hour fast once or twice a week. For example, if you stop eating at 8 p.m. on Saturday night, you wouldn't eat again until 8 p.m. on Sunday night.

Alternate day fasting

When following this method, you would eat in an ongoing cycle as follows: fast one day, eat normally the next, and so on. On fasting days, you would usually eat 500–600 calories.

However you choose to rest and renew your body through eating, try to stay away from high-sugar foods and drinks, as the insulin spike they will cause will probably make you want to eat more.

As always, if you are considering making changes that will affect how your body and its processes work, do your research, and give your doctor a heads-up. You are a grown-up and capable of making your own decisions. People with diabetes and those with unique digestive tracts may not benefit from fasting in any way, shape or form. Be smart.

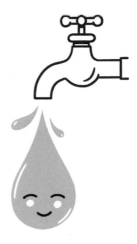

Hydro-homies

As a nurse, I've looked after many people who are experiencing dehydration: some because of neglect, others because they were too hot, others because they've forgotten to take water out with them on a hot day. Whatever the reason, dehydration can be rectified simply: by drinking.

When I was training, one of the things that I was taught over and over again is that hydration is important. People need water. It is one of the foundational chemicals that make our bodies work. If you go without water for seventy-two hours, your body starts to shut down and die.

Three days. That's it. What a morbid way to start a section.

"Water! You may not like it, but you have to drink it."

ANTHONY T. HINCKS

Now that I've (hopefully) impressed on you how important hydration is, I'm going to tell you why.

We are sixty per cent water. Our brains and hearts are composed of seventy-three per cent water. Our lungs are about eighty-three per cent water. Our skin contains sixty-four per cent water, our muscles and kidneys contain seventy-nine per cent. Even our bones are watery: thirty-one per cent. What I'm trying to say is, we are basically big bags of water with bits floating in them.

So, now I've told you just how sloshy you actually are, here are some things that water is used for in the body.

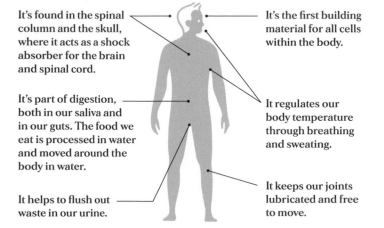

It's found in the spinal column and the skull, where it acts as a shock absorber for the brain and spinal cord.

It's the first building material for all cells within the body.

It's part of digestion, both in our saliva and in our guts. The food we eat is processed in water and moved around the body in water.

It regulates our body temperature through breathing and sweating.

It helps to flush out waste in our urine.

It keeps our joints lubricated and free to move.

When we don't get the water we need, our bodies cannot function correctly. This is called dehydration. If we experience dehydration, our super-clever bodies will stop doing non-essential things in order to keep us alive. We will stop digesting food; we'll stop making saliva; and our fingers and toes will get less water, as whatever water we have left in the body is kept in life-sustaining areas such as the head and the thorax. We will stop sweating and start to overheat. As our water content drops, so does our ability to process toxins. The more dehydrated we get, the more toxic we will become. Eventually, these toxic chemicals will build up in the brain, and we will find it hard to think and make good decisions. This does not allow us to rest well, as we feel rubbish and our bodies get stressed. Have you ever found it hard to think straight when you're hungover, or found yourself making bad decisions like eating rubbish food? That can be your toxic brain thinking.

DRINK UP

We adult humans need a MINIMUM of 2 litres (3½ pints) of water every day. Did you notice the capitalisation of MINIMUM? That means you can have more. Don't take it to extremes, of course, but drinking 4–5 litres (7–8½ pints) of water a day (in warm countries) will keep you super hydrated and peeing all the time.

It's important to note that your body can only take in so much water at a time. If you drink more than 250ml (just under ½ pint) in the space of fifteen minutes, your body can't process it and you will simply pee out the extra. Downing a pint every fifteen minutes will not be as effective as drinking lots of little sips throughout the day.

Putting water in your body is an instant way to relax: to change states, even for a second, because your body is having one of its core needs met and so does not have to worry for a while. Your unconscious mind knows you have enough water to survive for seventy two hours. So there is a worry gone from your unconcious.

Let's be clear here that I'm specifically talking about water. In the West, we are conditioned to like soda, cordial or other additives to water. In moderation, this is fine and good. When we look more closely at what is in those additives, though, it's easy to see how they might cause us some problems: caffeine makes us more dehydrated and can cause our bladders to spasm; sugar stimulates our nervous systems; artificial colours and preservatives cause our bodies to respond in a variety of different ways.

Drinking soda is great once in a while, but drinking it every day, or even as every drink, as some people do, can cause troubles far beyond simple dehydration. My recommendation: scrap the soda, get on the water.

ALCOHOL

If you are drinking alcohol, you are going to need to replenish your fluids as you go. Alcohol dehydrates you because it makes you pee (once you've broken the seal, right?) As a basic rule, for each unit of alcohol you drink, you need to drink 250 ml (about ½ pint) of water.

Good hydration

Hydration is one of the most effective and powerful forms of rest you can give your mind and body. When we are well hydrated, our body works efficiently: our organs are nicely suspended in fluid; our blood is the right consistency; we can digest effectively; and our faecal matter is nice and soft. Good hydration means that, when you sleep, the brain can effectively wash itself clean of the day's rubbish. Have you ever tried to wash wine glasses after you've washed a roasting tray in the sink? Not easy. It's the same for your brain: give it fresh water to help it clean up. And yes, downing a whole pint of water before bed will mean you wake up in the night needing to pee. Experiment: your body is uniquely beautiful. Find out how much to drink, and how long before bed you should drink it, so you can stay well hydrated without any night-time bathroom trips.

It's not just at night, either. Staying hydrated can improve your effectiveness throughout the day. I learned this as a nurse. On a busy shift, it can be hard to find the time to eat or drink, but this is faulty behaviour. I was almost surgically attached to my water bottle. Every opportunity I had, I'd drink: when I changed areas, when I used the computer, when I went to the supply room. I drank almost as often as I washed my hands. Engaging in the biological process of drinking changes your mental process. It breaks the pattern you are in, so you can move on to the next job effectively. Try it for yourself. Use your drinking water to change your mental state so you can be fresher for the next task. When you're finished in a meeting, drink your water before moving on to the next thing.

With adequate water in our systems, we are able dilute the toxins that our bodies produce naturally, allowing us to remove them without the negative effects they can cause, such as brain fog. You know when you get a cold or the flu, and you just want to lie in bed and quietly die? (Is that just a man thing?) If you drink water, lots of water, all the toxins from the infection are removed more easily, allowing you to heal faster. Your mucus will be runnier, allowing you to get rid of it more quickly, and your body will be more effective.

SMALL STEPS: RESTFUL HYDRATION

First things first – and I can't stress this enough. DRINK WATER.

Whether it's tap water (if it's safe to drink where you are) or bottled water (if your environmental ethics go that way), get that H_2O into your body.

Carrying a bottle or flask with you that you can refill is great: it cuts down on pollution. It can also help to find a water bottle that shows you how much you've drunk, so you can keep track and make sure you're staying hydrated.

If you don't have a funky water bottle that you can use to track your drinking, the old-fashioned way to check that you are hydrated is to look at your pee. If your urine is clear, or light yellow, you are on track for being hydrated. If it's darker, you need to drink more. If it's red, go see your doctor.

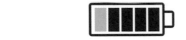

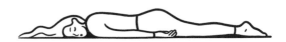

Recovering From Sleep Loss

"No Sleep Till Brooklyn"

THE BEASTIE BOYS

Entire books could be (and have been) written about sleep. Here, I'm going to talk specifically about how to rest to recover from sleep loss. When we miss sleep, our bodies and minds do not function as efficiently as they normally would. Whether you have a newborn baby, are too stressed or jet-lagged to sleep, or got up in the middle of the night to watch the fight, or in the case of the Beastie Boys, you have to fight for your right to party – whatever the reason, missing sleep means we don't function as well. Missing sleep is part of life, but with the advice in this section we are going to make it so we can excel even when little Timmy has woken us up at 3 a.m. by projectile vomiting.

Usually, broadly speaking, we sleep for seven to nine hours. Each person is different. If I don't get my nine hours, I am seriously grumpy, whereas my wife is good with six to seven hours. When we miss sleep, it means that the body has not had time to complete the cycles that it runs through at night. These cycles detox the body, store memories and process the things that we don't need. This is why new mums and dads often have what we call 'baby brain': broken and lost sleep has stopped their brains being able to effectively form new memories.

So, how can we make up for missed sleep? After all, life goes on and you can't just sit on the sofa and watch daytime TV in a daze after a sleepless night. I've got some tools for you.

Hydrate

I know we've just covered this in the Hydro-homies section (pages 105–111), but it's super important. Your cells require water and minerals to keep themselves functioning as best they can. When our bodies get stressed from poor or missed sleep, making your cells happier is a great way to feel better. When we have happy, well-hydrated cells, our bodies work better. You can also add minerals and vitamins to your water. I'm not saying you should chug sugary sports drinks, I'm saying you could try drinking a sugar-free one. The water in it will help you feel better, and the soluble minerals and vitamins will help your body function more effectively. This can help to lift the brain fog that comes with missed sleep, and they also help control the increased appetite we often experience after a sleepless night.

Build your immunity

Our immunity goes down when we miss sleep. To make sure our bodies are resting as well as possible, we need to look after them. As our immune function drops, the inflammatory response goes up. To help in restoring the functioning of your natural immunity, there are some supplements you can take. Supplements are, in my opinion, super important in today's commodified food economy, but don't take new ones unless you've spoken to a medical professional about your personal needs.

The first is activated charcoal. It's used in accident and emergency departments to soak up toxins in people who've taken things that are not agreeing with them. Activated charcoal will absorb any extra toxins in your digestive tract. (Please note that it can also make your stools black.)

Another is oregano oil, which you can get in tablet form or as gel capsules. Oregano oil is chock-full of antioxidants and works to help kill airborne germs.

To get the big guns out when helping your body restore after missed sleep, hit up the turmeric latte. Turmeric contains a compound called curcumin that provides an awesome boost for your immune system. If you are not based in hipster central, this is how you make a turmeric latte at home.

TURMERIC LATTE (Makes 2 servings)

- 300 ml (10 fl oz) coconut milk
- 100 ml (3½ fl oz) water
- 2 teaspoons coconut oil
- 1 teaspoon ground turmeric
- ¾ teaspoon ground ginger
- 1 teaspoon ground cinnamon
- honey or other sweetener of choice, to taste
- small pinch of Himalayan salt, or other salt
- carob or cocoa powder, for sprinkling (optional)

In a small saucepan over a medium heat, mix together the coconut milk and water and warm through. Just as the mixture starts to boil, take it off the heat.

Transfer the coconut milk mixture to a blender and add the coconut oil, turmeric, ginger, cinnamon, honey and salt.

Cover with the lid and blend for about 30 seconds.

Divide the turmeric latte between two cups and, if you like, sprinkle some carob or cocoa powder over the top. Enjoy your warming latte. This is especially good after you've been out drinking all night.

Caffeine

I know I've done it, I'm sure you have too. After not getting enough sleep, we hit all the caffeine. ALL THE CAFFEINE.

While this may seem like a great solution to your sleep-deprived brain, it's not always the most awesome idea. It might help you feel a bit better now, but too much caffeine will interfere with your next sleep pattern. The body takes about seven hours to process caffeine. So, that cup of coffee you drank at 6 p.m.? It's going to be in your system until 1 a.m.

You only need a couple of cups of coffee throughout the day to keep you going. Try to avoid the energy drinks and quadruple espressos.

Naptastic

You'll find my ultimate guide to napping on pages 137–141, but here we are specifically talking about how to use naps to restore yourself after not sleeping. For example, if you've only had three hours of sleep the night before because you rolled in at 4 a.m. and had to at work at 8 a.m., with a forty-minute commute. Of course, I have never done this.

But if you do find yourself in this position, your meagre three hours of sleep can be bolstered with three twenty-minute naps. They will restore the body as much as possible after all that missed sleep.

Movement

If you haven't slept, your body's metabolism is not what it needs to be. Your endocrine system won't function properly and your hormones won't be released as they should be. The best thing to do in this situation is to move. Get outside and get some sun on your face. This will activate your wake-up systems. Go for a twenty-minute walk outside so that your body realises it's daytime and you should be doing daytime stuff. Try doing some yoga or a few push-ups, too, as they will help reduce the anxiety that often comes with tiredness.

So, get moving and get the sun on your skin. If you do it before you eat, you will also increase your fat-burning abilities for the day.

Fuel

Our sleep cycle regulates our appetite. When we don't sleep properly, we often find we want to eat everything. This is because our levels of the hunger hormone, leptin, are going through the roof, while the hormone that makes us feel full, ghrelin, is nowhere to be found. Our instinct in this situation is to hit the carbs and fats – but don't. This will actually make you more tired, as they will mess with your insulin levels. The best way to fuel yourself when you are functioning on little sleep is to eat foods high in protein and low in fat and carbs. When we eat protein, our body releases a hormone called orexin, which keeps us awake. Basically, keep away from the burger and fries and grab yourself a Reuben on spelt.

RESTING TO REPAIR: RECAP

- How and what we eat and drink can help our bodies rest effectively.
- Our bodies can't digest effectively when we're stressed. Taking the time to practise gratitude before eating can help us move into Rest and Digest mode.
- Our bodies need water to function. Staying hydrated helps us rest and recover.
- We can use tools like hydration, exercise and napping to help our bodies recover after sleep loss.

05

Resting
to Renew

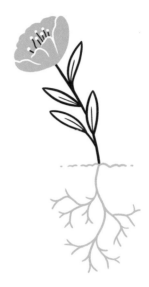

Inside & Out

Our cells are renewed daily. When we give our bodies the right conditions for our cells to renew in ways that are good and not unduly stressed, we stay healthy, fit and young. In the Ayurvedic model of health, being 'beautiful' means being healthy, not being covered in make-up or having perfectly styled hair. We're talking about internal, lustrous beauty that shines through – without concealer. This model of health, beauty and youthfulness brings renewal to your cells, and therefore to your entire body.

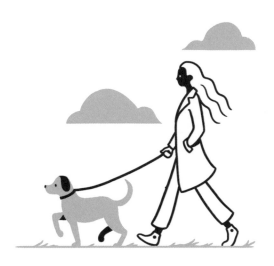

I Like to
Move it, Move it

"If we could give every individual the right amount of nourishment and exercise, not too little and not too much, we would have found the safest way to health."

HIPPOCRATES

As human beings, we are meant to move. We are *not* meant to sit in front of a computer screen or lie on the sofa watching TV all day (as much as I would like to).

In my role as a nurse, I once looked after a supercentenarian: a lady who lived past 110 years of age. One of the things she said helped her live so long was walking to the shops every day to get her shopping, then walking home: about two miles, every single day – and on Sunday, she walked to church. With her in mind, you and I have no excuse not to walk if we are able. On average, people who are healthy and reach the age of 100 or more have walked for up to five to six miles a day for most of their lives. (This was studied as part of the Blue Zone Project pioneered by Dan Buettner – for more on that, *radical-rest.com* has the links for you.)

In recent years, it has become common to believe that we should try and walk at least 10,000 steps a day. This concept actually originated with a Japanese company, Yamasa, who coincidentally manufactured pedometers. They chose the number 10,000 for branding reasons.

There are, however, some great benefits to walking 10,000 steps a day, which we'll explore. Everyone who has lived a long, healthy life has been physically active throughout their lives, and that movement continues into later life. Even when she was in hospital, my 110-year-old patient put in a good mile a day just by walking around the ward and talking to bed-bound people thirty or forty years younger than her.

When we walk, we create movement in our muscles. This muscle contraction activates and aids fluid drainage from our lower limbs. You know when you sit on a plane or train for ages and your legs swell up? This is because you are not walking, and aiding fluid drainage. This helps your circulation and soothes your nervous system, and the impact force of your feet meeting the floor makes your bones stronger, reducing the chance of brittle bones in later life. It's a whole-body workout that is nourishing and supportive to the renewal process. Walking is also a great way to take yourself away from the 'noise' of your life and renew yourself in nature. It's not just good for your body: it benefits your mind, too.

RENEWAL THROUGH MOVEMENT

You know the drill. Try to walk 10,000 steps every day. Ten thousand steps might be the goal, BUT – and I need to stress this – if you spend most of your day sitting, whether that's at a desk or in a vehicle, or on the sofa, any amount of movement is a win.

Look at how you can change your work life to help you move more. Things like standing desks or walking desks can help. If your boss has a budget for these adaptions, encourage them to use it. If not, look at other ways of adding dynamic movements to your day.

Our bodies are designed to walk, to move. This is a very basic biological model of health: when we don't move, our bodies go wrong.

FLUID

When we don't move, walk, dance, etc., our bodies can't return the fluid from our extremities back to our hearts as effectively. When you walk, the muscles in your calves, thighs and butt contract and relax to move you forward. At the same time, the muscles in your core are working to keep you from falling over. This contraction and relaxation of muscles brings fluid from your feet and back up to your body for processing.

If you don't move around, your lack of movement can put a strain on your heart because your heart is having to work harder to bring that fluid up the body, without the accessory muscles helping. When we are inactive, our hearts have to work harder to move blood from our feet back up to our hearts. This strain ages your heart, and is not restful. If you keep your body moving, you will put less strain on your heart. (It will also stop you from getting cankles, so win-win.)

HORMONES

Hormones are an awesome support when it comes to movement. You don't have to lift heavy weights or get your CrossFit on: simply walking can give you a great hormone hit. When we move in easy, gentle ways (and remember, everyone's 'easy' is different), the body's natural ability to remove oxidative compounds from itself comes into play. As our muscles move, anti-inflammatory hormones are released to stop the muscles swelling due to damage in the right now, the acute. One of these hormones is glucagon. Glucagon is also part of the mechanism that controls sugar in the body. When your muscles burn through their sugar reserves, glucagon gets the body to release the additional sugar that the muscles need to move. This double effect helps to make sure the muscles are well-fed, as well as controlling the immediate swelling. Have you ever noticed that when you are in the gym, you don't look as pumped as you do twenty minutes later? This is because while you're actually working out, your muscles are full of blood fuelling them, and the swelling is controlled. When you are done in the gym and are slurping your protein shake, your guns get bigger, right? The acute phase has passed, and other things need to happen to make sure your muscles are fuelled and healed.

This means that, by exercising, you de-stress your body, using its natural processes to remove the oxidative molecules that cause stress (antioxidants – see page 54 and 55). This gentle movement and release of hormones also helps release endorphins. Endorphins rock. These happy hormones help you relax and chill while feeling good.

This management of hormones through exercise is a great way to increase your ability to rest, as your body is doing what it is supposed to do. The act of resting through movement is about putting your body into the state it has evolved to be in. When we allow our bodies to behave in the ways in which they have evolved to behave, they are much more efficient at dealing with all the things life throws at us.

MOOD

As you move your body, you start to allow your whole physiology to rest effectively and become more stress-free. You allow your nervous system to drop back into Rest and Digest mode. This has the added bonus of improving your mood.

By moving your body, you allow your conscious mind to focus on the movements you are making rather than the thoughts you are having. If you are trying to hit a ball with a bat or put your feet in the right places for the dance you're trying to do, you can't focus on the problem that has been worrying you or bringing you down. This is not about dismissing that thought pattern, but about changing the focus for a brief time to give your mind a chance to rest. This resting through movement allows your mind to temporarily reprogramme, so it's not constantly focused on anxiety or depression. The more you do this, the easier it is to forget your unhelpful thought patterns. This is because your conscious brain is only really any good at focusing on one thing at a time, so when you are focusing on the position of your feet, or where the ball is, or what your lungs are doing, your brain hasn't got the bandwidth to also worry about whatever problem has been bothering you.

In this way, you can use movement to rest your overactive mind and reprogramme yourself to behave differently.

SMALL STEPS: MOVEMENT

Start within your comfort zone and build up. If walking 10,000 steps seems impossible, remember that walking 100 steps is still lapping everyone who is just sitting on the sofa. And it doesn't have to be walking – you could choose to dance, or do yoga, or walk on your hands. Choose the movement that suits you. By adding gentle movement to your everyday life, you allow your body to rest, your mind to process and your spirits to soar.

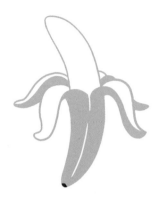

Get Your Freak On

"An orgasm a day keeps the doctor away."

THE NHS

This is a fun one. To rest your endocrine system, specifically your reproductive hormones, orgasms are your friend. Yup, orgasms. They are good for you, on many levels. (Not just the obvious ones.)

One of the needs our primitive brain has is the need to reproduce. Our programming is designed to make sure our genes survive by being passed forward to the next generation. When we have an orgasm, our primitive brain thinks we have achieved the goal of reproducing. Even though, in our modern world, the need to reproduce may feel less urgent, this does not stop our primitive brain getting antsy if we don't orgasm often enough.

When we orgasm, a whole range of feel-good chemicals are released. For guys it's oxytocin, testosterone, dopamine and vasopressin; while the ladies get a big ol' dose of oxytocin, dopamine, testosterone and endorphins. The bigger the orgasm, the more oxytocin gets released, and the happier and more relaxed you feel. Women win this game as, post-orgasm, guys also get a big dose of vasopressin, which uses up all the neurotransmitters that allow orgasm. Women don't get that: they get to go on and have multiple orgasms, releasing yet more of the happy hormones.

The more you know, eh?

So, why am I talking about orgasms and rest? It's all about pacifying the primative part of your brain so you don't feel stressed out, on a deep, unconscious level, about procreation. Having an orgasm (or six) helps to manage your body's *perception* of reproducing, which reduces that unconscious stress and releases the good hormones that help us relax. It's all about hormone and neurotransmitter management. You can utilise your biology at root level to help you relax on a radical level.

In women who are perimenopausal, having an orgasm at least once a month can move back the start of menopause. This is pretty awesome news in this world of push, push, push, where women are pressured to achieve more and more professionally and then have kids. Getting help with having an orgasm is even more effective than solo fun at pushing back the start of menopause. I suggest that multiple orgasms are the best way forward, just to be sure – you know, for science. These orgasms don't have to involve a penis in order to extend your fertile years: in fact, dual clitoral and vaginal stimulation is more effective than just vaginal orgasms for this purpose. Plus, women are probably more likely to know where their own clitoris is. Just saying. However you choose to do it, this way of resting allows the body to release the hormones that are required to keep you fertile. This means that, by actively seeking orgasms, you are resting your body and allowing it to do what it was designed to do on a genetic level.

For men, it's suggested that, in order to help reduce the risk of prostate cancer, you need to orgasm at least once a week. Again, this orgasm can be achieved alone or with a friend – it's up to you. For men, orgasm can clear the urethral tract and stimulate the prostate so it does not atrophy or start to go wrong. This form of rest allows your body to restore itself and keep healthy – that's what rest is all about, right?

In your early twenties, having lots of sex can help to set up your body for longevity. Your body responds better to all sorts of stresses, as long as you are having sex. And not just orgasms. The human interaction that comes with sex – the play, the arousal, the fun – builds stronger resilience against stress, both on a neurological and an immune system level.

SMALL STEPS: REST AND RENEWAL THROUGH SEX
Have orgasms. Many and varied. If you don't know how, the internet is full of instructional videos. You do you. Literally.

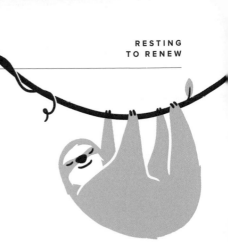

The Power of Napping

"I can't get no sleep, I need to sleep."

FAITHLESS

I love a nap. In fact, I've just had one.

Naps are a great way to resolve accumulated sleep loss. Unless I'm working at the hospital, when it's not always possible, I like to take a twenty-minute nap every day, usually after lunch.

There is some science behind my early afternoon snooze. A thirty-minute nap has been shown to increase performance in speed trials (when you race a car or bike for a long period to see how it lasts). From this, we can infer that a nap helps us use the energy in our bodies more effectively. Even better, post-nap, our motor skills are improved, our memories are sharper and we are more resilient against injury. Naps can also reduce high blood pressure and improve our heart health. What's not to love?

A word of warning, though. Poorly timed naps, for example in the afternoon or evening, can cause insomnia. Timing does really matter.

How to nap

1. Don't use an alarm clock. Our brains work like a computer. When we snooze, our memories are transferred from the random-access memory to the hard drive. We sleep in stages. During light sleep, our memories are moved from the thinking part of our brain. When we go into rapid eye movement (REM) sleep, these memories get stored in our memory banks. This happens during cycles, which take about ninety minutes. When we nap, this process starts to happen: the memories are sorted, but not stored. When we wake up because of an alarm, the process gets interrupted and our memories can be half in our thinking brain and half in our memory. This makes memories harder to find – they can even be lost. When we allow ourselves to wake up naturally, this doesn't happen, as the brain stores the information where it knows it can find it. Being woken by a sudden alarm also delivers a jolt of adrenaline and cortisol, both unneeded hormones when we are trying to chill.

When you first start napping, try it at a time when you don't need to worry about oversleeping, like at home at the weekend. Then train yourself, over time, to wake up from a nap after thirty minutes to one hour. To give yourself this experience, start by napping at a time and in a place where it won't matter if you sleep for too long, like just after lunch at home on a Saturday. Not at your desk in the office at three o'clock in the afternoon on a Thursday. Practice makes perfect. Being clothed, hydrated and having noise around you helps your unconscious mind know this is just a twenty-minute refresh, not an eight-hour slumber party. If you do have to use an alarm clock, choose one that wakes you up gently. There are apps and different kinds of clocks that can do this. The more you practise napping, the better you will become at giving yourself the time you need and waking up naturally.

2. Schedule your nap. Our bodies respond best to a nap about seven hours after we wake up in the morning. I get up at 6 a.m., so 1 p.m. works well for me. The ideal times for your nap are usually between 11 a.m. and 3 p.m.

3. Don't drink caffeinated drinks before your nap. The whole point of taking a nap is to rest. The myth that coffee metabolises into your system to wake you up is not true, as even the tiny amount of caffeine absorbed through your mouth and throat is enough to inhibit your sleep quality. Plus, if you are napping in the afternoon, having caffeine that late in the day can mess with your sleep. You can have your morning coffee but having a big ol' cup of joe with lunch and expecting to have a meaningful nap is just a waste of that awesome caffeine. A glass of water would do just as well.

4. Pay attention to how long you nap for. If your naps are super long, it's a sign you need get more sleep at night. The naps we're talking about here are not intended to make up for missed sleep; they are to aid your body in processing and renewing itself. If you find your naps getting longer and longer, it's a good sign you need to go to bed earlier or look at your sleep hygiene.

5. Avoid stress before your nap. This is all about scheduling. Try to plan the low-stress things you do during the day for just before your nap: things like household chores, tidying your desk or eating lunch. Definitely not sending important emails or consulting with clients.

6. Don't exercise just before your nap. You need a minimum of forty-five minutes to chill out after exercising to get the full regenerative benefits of a nap.

7. Eat before you nap. Don't nap hungry, as low blood sugar will impair the quality; post-lunch is the best time for your nap. Your body will use the food in your gut to repair and renew itself as you doze.

8. Don't force it. Like orgasms and perfect ponytails, you can't force a nap. If it's not for you, no problem.

9. Make it a habit. Our brains love a pathway, a habit. Building yourself a pre-nap ritual is important. This is so your brain knows that, when you do the pre-nap ritual, you are going to sleep for thirty minutes and wake up. Perform the same sequence of activities every day, and lie down in the same position, at same time.

10. Don't use alcohol or sleeping tablets to start your nap. If you
have wine with your lunch, your nap will leave you groggy, sluggish
and fatigued.

To make this easy for you, there are Radical Rest Yoga Nidras
(guided meditative relaxation practices) available at *radical-rest.com*
that you can download. These are guided meditations that guide
you into a deeply relaxed state and through the process of the nap
cycle to wake you up at the end. These meditations are free for you
– you deserve it.

EYE MASKS

Depending on the amount of light pollution in your life, eye
masks may be the way forward when you nap or sleep. They
help reduce the amount of stimulation you get from light when
you are napping or asleep. Great for a post-lunch snooze.

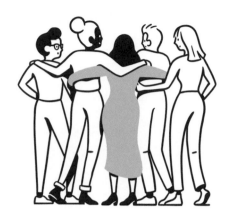

Society's Darling

"We don't heal in isolation, but in community."

S. KELLEY HARRELL

Remember the 110-year-old I met in hospital? She was literally the life and soul of the party. Some of my patients didn't see anyone beyond the nursing team from day to day. She, on the other hand, had multiple visitors. When at home, she was hosting dinner parties or going out with friends.

All. The. Time.

She loved to talk and listen and she was as sharp as a pin, despite having lived decades longer than people old enough to be her children.

As humans, we need social interaction to keep us healthy in mind, body and spirit. Socialising – spending time with friends, engaging in something fun – allows our brains to stop overthinking, and our bodies to get their primitive needs met. The ability to rest ourselves by being social is all about mitigating the stresses that build up when we don't get our basic needs met.

The need for human interaction

Let's think back to Maslow's hierarchy of needs in chapter one. One of the things that Maslow included in his hierarchy was human interaction. We need to be around other humans. Something that the 2020 coronavirus pandemic has shown us was that humans will go out of their way, even in the face of potential death, to be near those who they count as their family or their clan. Even though some countries were literally paying people to stay at home, like the UK and Italy, some people would risk themselves and others in order to be social. Large parts of the US even had armed protests about being forced to isolate. This desire to be social is a vital part of being a human, and when we deny it, we get stressed. And, remember: stress does not equal good rest.

Our primitive brain, the super ancient neurology likes to socialise because, when we are around other humans in a social way, we release oxytocin, a hormone that helps us to relax. Oxytocin is especially released when we hug. We have evolved to be social creatures and to see our mutual survival as dependent on those around us. When we look at other mammals in their herds or family groups, we can see that they often have one or two members watching for predators, so the rest can feel safe and rest, feed, drink, etc. This behaviour is wired into us as mammals on a very primitive level: that we need to be in a group to survive. Harking back to the 2020 pandemic again, the people who suffered most were those who lived alone, away from their social group. When we are alone, our primitive neurology thinks it is in danger and isolated, and so there is an increased likelihood of being eaten. This stresses the body, meaning full rest is harder to come by.

Trust and respect

There has got to be trust and respect in your social group, whether it's a club you are part of or friends you've known since college. In my time as a nurse in the accident and emergency department, I saw many groups of friends come in, usually because one of them had taken too much or drunk too much. Of course, the mate who'd ended up hospitalised was often mocked, and silly photos were taken, but that is just friendship tax. The important thing was the group was there to look after their sick friend. These friends are the ones you want; not the small but very real minority who'd call an ambulance for their passed-out friend and leave them on the pavement, so as not to spoil their own night. There is no trust there. If, in your most vulnerable moment, you can't trust your friends to help, they are not your friends.

It was noted in a study in Edinburgh that people's immune and inflammatory response changed when they were with friends they trusted. For example, the immune response to viruses like the cold virus was higher, but the inflammatory response was less. This means your body gets measurably less stressed when you are with people you trust, and also more resistant to infection.

Digital society is OK, but it's like having a glass of water when you actually want a glass of wine, or watching a film about the beach instead of actually going to the beach. It keeps you going, but the experience is not the same. We don't get the full gamut of hormone release that comes with being in physical proximity to other humans. In real life, when we hang out with our friends, our body can read other bodies, our hormones respond to theirs and our immune response gets better. We get better. Our bodies become less stressed, and we're able to rest, relax and renew.

To allow ourselves to rest our social primitive ancient mammalian brain, and reduce our stress levels, we can try to make sure that we meet and interact with other humans, be they family, friends, co-workers, or people you see in a club or hobby group.

SMALL STEPS: SOCIALISING FOR REST AND RENEWAL
Hang out with people who you respect and trust, and who respect and trust you back: people who you feel safe around.

If you don't have many friends in your area, join a club, sports team or society. Reach out to a club or group you are interested in, and then actually turn up. It can be photography, football, archery, Dungeons and Dragons, tree-hugging, yoga – whatever tickles your pickle. Go and find like-minded humans and make oxytocin together.

REST FOR RENEWAL: RECAP

◆ As human beings, we're designed to move. Whether you walk, dance or do yoga, regular physical activity will help keep your body working as it should, releasing the right hormones and reducing stress. Focusing on a physical activity also enables our minds to rest.

◆ We evolved to procreate. Having regular orgasms satisfies this primitive need and releases happy hormones.

◆ A short nap every day can help us feel more energetic and focused.

◆ Social interaction with people we trust satisfies a key part of our primitive 'monkey brain' and makes us feel safe, helping us to rest effectively.

06

·

Resting
for Resilience

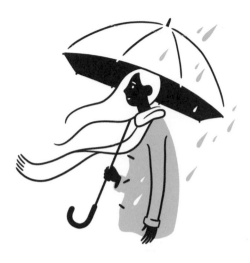

Decoding
Your Body

Resting for resilience is a way of pre-resting your body to allow you to cope with whatever life throws at you. Our original settings are those of hunter-gatherers who roamed the land looking for food, water and shelter. We can access these settings with relative ease (it's not always pleasant, mind you, but it is quite easy). The practices in this chapter will help you unlock and decode the core parts of your body and mind that are dormant and just waiting for you to access them.

When we reach inside ourselves and find that the resilience we need to cope with any situation is already there, we can begin to realise that we are pretty powerful beings. It helps us to remember who we are and to trust ourselves, rather than looking elsewhere for information and validation.

When we allow other influences to affect our personal worldview, we can start to develop interesting (not always in a good way) patterns and beliefs about ourselves. These new less-than-optimal patterns and beliefs go against how we have evolved to be. When we go against our own DNA, our own physicality, we become stressed, and when we are stressed, we can't rest. I'm going to say, right now, that this is not our fault. Our society is set up to hypnotise us to feel less-than-good about ourselves in order to sell us things. This is part of the societal hypnosis I talked about earlier (pages 18 and 19). While it's not our fault, it is most definitely our responsibility to sort it out within ourselves.

By using rest to access our most basic settings and find the resilience within ourselves, we can become the humans we are supposed to be, without the negative influence of societal hypnosis trying to make us believe that we are not good enough. By doing this, we are allowing some of the conditioning of the world to slide off, leaving us as just us. Like, totally us. This is a great thing to be able to do after a long day at work when you are about to go on a date or hang out with friends.

We are going to utilise your ability to rest and develop resilience in order to maximise your time and energy. We've all heard the saying that a change is as good as a rest. Well, it's actually true, but a rest is always my first option.

Our bodies go through a lot. They are supremely adapted to keep us alive and functioning and can survive even the most hideous injuries: my nursing career has taught me that. From everyday bumps and bruises to sickness, disease and bad sushi, our bodies will always fight to stay alive, to heal and to restore.

The problem is, our modern lives tend not to give us time to let our bodies restore. Will your boss give you a day off if you've got a cold? Can you give yourself time off when you have a cold? Do parents *ever* get time off? We don't give ourselves time to heal or space to rest.

Our bodies are pretty primitive things: we've established that. They are, however, filled with a load of cool processes and abilities that we rarely activate, as we've made very comfortable lives for ourselves. To restore our bodies and minds, we are going to learn how to use some of them. This allows us to rest, even when things are getting out of hand. Let's look at how we can help the body to restore itself using some ancient techniques that are also backed up by cutting-edge science.

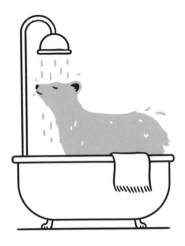

Ice, Ice, Baby

The Vikings did it; yoga gurus recommend it; in Scandinavia, it's practically a religion. It is the ancient and nipple-hardening art of ice baths. A Dutch guy by the name of Wim Hoff brought this technique to the eyes of the wider world. Wim is known as 'the Ice Man'. He performs amazing feats of cold endurance, like swimming in the Antarctic. Wim and his team of scientists discovered that the way these practices have conditioned and hardened his body's systems – the nervous system, the endocrine system and everything else – has left both his mind and body incredibly resilient to stress. His methods have even made him more resistant to infections: he cured himself from toxins injected straight into his body just by using his techniques.

"Before competition, I always take an ice bath to make my body feel more refreshed. Then I always have coffee with a little cream and sugar. It's a superstitious thing."

MCKAYLA MARONEY

What is good about the tools and techniques that Wim teaches is that they are not limited to him; they can be learned by we regular people. To help your body to rest effectively in a world that is more stressful than we'd like, I want you to harden your immune and nervous systems. But how? Can you see where I'm going here?

Take a breath. I'm not going to ask you to take an ice bath. I can feel your cortisol rising from here.

If you are not quite as used to being in freezing waters as the Finns or Norwegians, never fear. There is a less intense way of doing it, that gives you similar benefits without having to fight off polar bears. (If, however, you do want to go to the Fjords and try it out, rock on.)

I'm going to tell you how to use the same techniques in your shower. Much easier, less bitey, with considerably fewer icebergs.

When we take a cold shower, our bodies respond. They respond first by asking 'WTF, brain? Why are you doing this to me?!'. Then they start to get stressed. I've waxed lyrical about *reducing* stress so far, so bear with me (*bear* with me, see what I did there?). This cold stress is a super-primal form of stress that our bodies have a genetic neurological pathway for coping with. At some time, all of our ancestors had to cope with being cold. The pathway that is activated here allows us to not only survive being cold, but to actually thrive because of it.

When we are exposed to cold in this way, our bodies start to release stress hormones and increase the speed of our breathing. What happens next is the cool part (ha! Pun-tastic). When we turn off the cold shower and start to warm up, our bodies calm down. When repeated, this process is called stress hardening, and it makes our bodies more resilient to *all* forms of stress. This stress hardening is what helps your body remain calm when everything's going wrong.

Taking a cold shower also makes us become naturally more alert. The cold stimulates the nervous system into taking deep breaths, lowering the carbon dioxide in the body, making it easier for us to concentrate. This result persists throughout the day. You don't need to pop off for a cold shower every few hours.

Even better, when we are exposed to the cold, our bodies respond by making more white blood cells. These are the cells that kill infections and protect against disease. By training your body to endure the cold of the shower, you also train your immune response and nervous system to respond differently. You harden them. This means your body will be able to attack and overwhelm some infections, viruses, bacteria or toxins in short order, whereas other people will get sick.

What more can this process give? Well, the simple fact of standing in a cold shower for extended periods is not pleasant, and training yourself to do it every day builds neurological pathways around willpower. The more you force yourself into the cold shower, the stronger your willpower becomes. Again, this is restoring your body to its natural settings.

These cold showers can also help with weight loss. During repetitive exposure to cold showers, our bodies use up brown fat. This brown fat is what is burned for quick energy: we get cold and burn off our energy stores. Brown fat is different to white fat. White fat is what we see in muffin tops or moobs; it is bulky and bad for us. The more we practise cold showers, the more our bodies repurpose white fat into brown fat, which is a good thing. The increase in metabolism that comes from having cold showers also burns off still more white fat. It's also good to note that brown fat is actually super good for you. We don't have loads of it, but when we do have it, it's a great form of easy-access energy.

SMALL STEPS: STRESS HARDENING

I know you are super excited to get started and jump in that cold shower. Who wouldn't be?

It's important, though, that you don't start by just having the coldest shower ever. It will shock you and you won't do it again. Here is the method I use.

First, have a nice, warm shower and wash yourself like normal.

Now, hold the showerhead in your hand, pointing away from you, and turn the water temperature down. You don't need it to be icy cold: 15°C (60°F) is cold enough.

Slowly let the cold water run over you, starting with your feet, then your legs and arms, before moving on to the rest of your body. Starting with your extremities like this helps to get your body used to what's going on.

Now shower your whole body in the cold water for fifteen seconds. Count fifteen 'Mississippis', then jump out. Turn the shower off (and remember to reset the temperature to warm: whoever uses it next will thank you).

Do this for a week. The following week, increase your time by fifteen seconds. Keep adding fifteen seconds each week for the next month, until you are taking a minute-long cold shower. You can then choose to lower the temperature or add more time: but don't do both at once. Be kind to yourself. A couple of minutes is the maximum you need (unless you enjoy it, in which case, rock on). This technique builds the stress hardening you need to be more resilient against the stresses of the world around us.

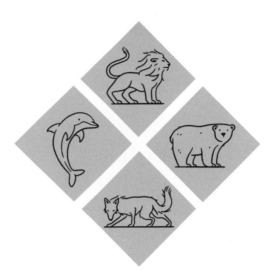

Understanding
Your Chronotype

Your chronotype is based on the timing of your personal biology.
This is the work of an awesome guy called Michael Breus. He is
known as America's Sleep Doctor, and more in-depth information on
chronotypes can be found in his book *The Power of When*.

I want you to know about your chronotype so that you can find the
most optimal way to rest and restore yourself throughout the day.
When we work with our own biological set-up rather than against it,

we can rest much more effectively. This is only a guide; I advise using the type that fits your world about eighty per cent of the time. That way, you can get a good fit without worrying about fitting perfectly.

"I don't believe in a chronological way of doing things."

YOKO ONO

There are four chronotypes.

 DOLPHIN: About ten per cent of the population are dolphins. Dolphins are light sleepers and are often misdiagnosed as insomniacs.

Dolphin day plan

6.30am	Get up and move
7.30am	Breakfast
9.30am	Coffee time
10am – 12pm	Be creative and conceptualise
12pm	Eat lunch
1pm – 4pm	Light exercise (or a walk if you're feeling tired)
4pm – 6pm	Time for the hard mental work
6pm	Practise yoga, meditate, pray
6.30pm – 8pm	Dinner
10.30pm	Turn all tech off
11.30pm	Bedtime

LION: About twenty per cent of the population are lions. Lions are early risers and wake up full of energy, but they run out by the end of the day.

Lion day plan

5.30am	Wake up and have breakfast
6am – 7am	Plan your day/world domination
9am – 10am	Coffee
10am – 12pm	Be sociable and interact with people. This is the best time for you to schedule meetings.
12pm	Eat lunch
1pm – 5pm	Do creative, inspirational work
5pm– 6pm	Move your body
6pm – 7pm	Eat dinner
10pm	Turn all tech off
10.30pm	Bedtime

 BEARS: Bears make up about fifty per cent of the population. They work with the sunset and sunrise, and like eight hours of sleep.

Bear day plan

7am	Wake up and move your body
7.30am	Eat breakfast
9am – 10am	Organise your life
10am	Coffee
10am – 12pm	Now is the time to complete hard mental tasks and be professional

Bear day plan

12pm	Move, eat lunch, move again
2.30pm – 3pm	Nap
3pm – 6pm	Social time. Try to schedule meetings for this time
6pm – 7pm	Move your body again
7.30pm	Eat dinner
8pm – 10pm	Conceptualise and plan tomorrow
10pm	All tech off
11pm	Go to sleep

 WOLVES: Wolves make up about twenty per cent of the population. They are not early risers; they are the life and soul at night.

Wolf day plan

7am	Use all the alarms to wake up, then journal. Wolves need the alarms, you need that jolt to get you out of bed.
7.30am	Eat breakfast
8.30am	Go outside and move
9am	Organise your life
11am – 1pm	Do the chores, drink coffee
1pm	Head outside for a walk and eat something
4pm – 6pm	This is your most social time, so schedule meetings for now. Be a human being
6pm – 7pm	Move your body
8pm	Eat dinner
11pm	All tech off
12pm	Go to bed

These chronotypes are not here for you to beat yourself up with. They are presented so you can see how your body works and understand that everybody works differently. This makes sense: as a cave person, you would have lived with others who had different chronotypes to you to make sure you were all safe overnight and during the day, as different members of your group would be more alert at different times.

We can use this information to make sure that we are not forcing ourselves to conform to schedules or routines that make us grumpy or stressed. Instead, we can use these chronotypes to help us understand how best to rest, to utilise our inner programming on a genetic level. This will make us more productive at work, and in life generally.

DON'T BE ALARMED
When we are woken by a jarring noise, like an alarm or someone banging on the door, our bodies go from a restful state to full-blown Fight or Flight, instantly stressing us out. Change your life for the better by assigning a pleasant noise for your alarm, like bird song or a music track that gradually gets louder.

REST FOR RESILIENCE: RECAP

- ◆ We can find ways to tap into our original hunter-gatherer settings, enabling us to become more resilient to stress.
- ◆ The cold shower stress-hardening technique is a powerful way of boosting our resilience and helps us handle stress more effectively.
- ◆ Understanding your chronotype can help you work out how best to plan your day to suit your own personal biology.

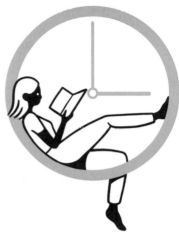

Conclusion: Start Your Rest Revolution

A call to action

I want for you to be the best, most rested you possible. This means having to take radical responsibility for yourself: for how you act, how your body works and how your mind works. That's hard to do in a culture that tries to make us conform and stay small. You were not born to conform. You were born to excel; billions of years of evolution have told us that. We have evolved to be able to prosper and live a fulfilled life in the world. This book is full of loads of different tools and techniques; take the ones that work for you and tweak and adapt them to make them uniquely yours.

* Nap during your lunch break.
* Dance after meetings. Or before, or during, or all three.
* Hug a friend.
* Drink some water.
* Have some coffee.
* Have a cold shower.
* Smell nice smells.
* Set goals.

Rest your body in the way that you want to rest it.

When you notice that you are getting stressed, anxious or depressed, take yourself out of the situation and practise your deep breaths. When you have returned to a place of balance, begin again. You have the power. Use it.

About the Author

Richard Lister is a trained nurse, educator, coach, meditation practitioner, yoga teacher, Ayurvedic therapist, massage therapist, author, educator, public speaker, fire walking instructor and all-round awesome human.

He's worked with people in clinical and domestic settings since the early 2000s, and is passionate about self-determination and using the skills that you have within you to become the best-ever version of yourself.

He chose to leave nursing when he had a breakdown from the sheer volume of human suffering that he encountered, alongside not having good coping strategies. That's why he developed Radical Rest and the umbrella practice of Medicine for Modern Times.

Further Reading

All the references and evidence that is book is based on can be found at **radical-rest.com**

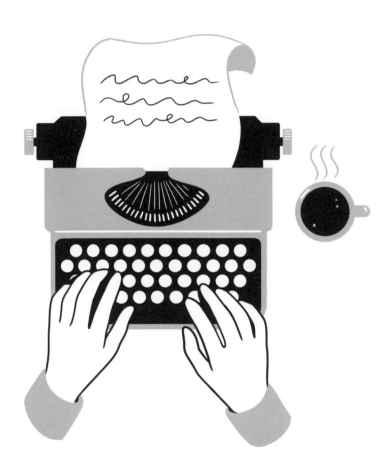

Index

Published in 2021 by Hardie Grant Books,
an imprint of Hardie Grant Publishing

Hardie Grant Books (London)
5th & 6th Floors
52–54 Southwark Street
London SE1 1UN

Hardie Grant Books (Melbourne)
Building 1, 658 Church Street
Richmond, Victoria 3121

hardiegrantbooks.com

British Library Cataloguing-in-Publication Data. A catalogue record
for this book is available from the British Library.

Radical Rest by Richard Lister

ISBN: 978-1-78488-377-5

10 9 8 7 6 5 4 3 2 1

Publisher: Kajal Mistry
Editor: Eve Marleau
Design and Illustration: Julia Murray
Copy-editor: Tara O'Sullivan
Proofreader: Gregor Shepherd
Indexer: Vanessa Bird
Production Controller: Sinead Hering

Colour reproduction by p2d
Printed and bound in China by Leo Paper Products Ltd.

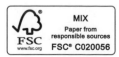

MIX
Paper from
responsible sources
FSC
www.fsc.org   FSC® C020056